Contents

Acknowledgements

I am indebted to the authors of the chapters of this book. It has been a privilege to commission, liaise and sometimes harass such a dedicated group of people. I have learnt something new from each chapter; whether increasing my understanding of what is happening overseas, being introduced to approaches that are novel to me, or reflecting on my own approach to supervision. In order of appearance:

Don Brand, Caroline Webb, John Carpenter, Marion Bogo, Jane Paterson, Allyson Davys, Liz Beddoe, Tish Marrable, Sharon Lambley, Jane Wonnacott, Sonya Wallbank, Andy Bradley, Rhiannon Barker, Esther Flanagan, Jeremy Winter, Kevin Brett, Maryam Zonouzi and Paul Ross.

I am very grateful that they have made the time to contribute to this book, despite the many demands that they face. They have been enthusiastic, supportive and responsive to my suggestions and editorial changes, thank you.

I am also very grateful to the commissioning editor at Pavilion, Jan Alcoe. Thank you for realising my potential and giving me this opportunity to suggest this collection. I would also like to acknowledge Ruth Chalmers for her patience and careful editing, and Helen Charlton for ensuring the book gets the best possible conference launch.

My friends and former colleagues from SCIE, Don Brand, Marie Diggins and Paul Ross, have repeatedly listened, advised and even provided the odd bit of pedantic grammatical advice!

A final thank you to my little boys, Isaac and Atticus. They live in the moment and remind me that while interprofessional supervision is important, at home, you can't beat a bit of junk modeling, whether making a Shard from shiny paper or the London Eye from an old tissue box and a paper plate!

About the contributors

Lyn Romeo

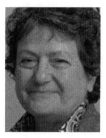

Lyn Romeo took up her post as chief social worker for adults in September 2013. Previously, Lyn worked as the assistant director for adult social care in the London Borough of Camden. She has also worked as an inspector with the Social Services Inspectorate, as well as working in Yorkshire for over 20 years as both a field social worker and in a variety of management roles across children and adults.[1]

Dr Lisa Bostock

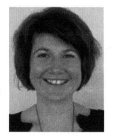

Lisa Bostock is an experienced social researcher, specialising in integrated working. Unusually, Lisa has worked across housing, health and social care, children's and adult social care and in different countries, Britain and Australia. She has worked in both the academic and non-government sector.

Lisa currently works at The Tilda Goldberg Centre for Social Work and Social Care, University of Bedfordshire. She manages two major evaluations within the Department for Education (DfE) children's social care innovation programme: implementation of the 'reclaiming social work' approach in five local authorities (Derbyshire, Harrow, Hull, Southwark and Buckinghamshire) and the redesign of the family safeguarding services in Hertfordshire.

Prior to joining TGC, Lisa worked at the Social Care Institute for Excellence (SCIE) for 11 years. At SCIE, Lisa led a programme of work on integration, including commissioning and co-authoring a major review of effective supervision that provided the impetus for this book.

She has published academic papers in the following peer review journals: *Children and Society, Children and Youth Services Review, Health and Social Care in the Community, Journal of Integrated Care, Sociology of Health and Illness* and *Social Science and Medicine.*

---

1 Parliament.uk, 2015. © Parliamentary copyright. Contains public sector information licensed under the Open Government License v3.0. To view this document, visit www.nationalarchives.gov.uk/doc/open-governement-licence/

Don Brand MBE

Don qualified as a social worker in 1969. After 20 years in Oxford and Kent social services departments, where he also helped to set up MCCH, a third sector provider of community housing, care and support services for people leaving the long-stay hospitals, he became deputy chief inspector in the Department of Health's social services inspectorate. Moving in 1996 to the National Institute for Social Work (NISW), he was involved with setting up the four UK Social Care Councils, the Topss England National Training Organisation, and the Social Care Institute for Excellence (SCIE). He has worked with SCIE, the College of Social Work and other national social care bodies, user-led organisations, government departments, the Law Commission and the devolved administrations. He is a trustee of the Joseph Rowntree Foundation and the Residential Forum.

Caroline Webb

Caroline is a qualified social worker specialising in social work with children and families, and is a current PhD candidate at the University of Bristol supervised by Professor John Carpenter.

She is particularly interested in issues relating to the social work workforce, and is currently working with Research in Practice (RiP) as part of a team leading a 'Change Project' on Reflective Supervision. Caroline has also worked with the Social Care Institute for Excellence (SCIE) to co-author a research briefing on 'Effective Supervision in Social Work and Social Care'.

Co-authored with colleagues, her latest research publications include an article in the *British Journal of Social Work* which systematically reviewed strategies for promoting the retention of social workers, and a paper published in *Children & Youth Services Review* highlighting the 'surprisingly weak' evidence base for supervision.

Caroline has also recently completed an MSc in social work research methods at the University of Bristol, and also holds an MSc in social work and a BSc in psychology.

Professor John Carpenter

Over the last 15 years John has carried out research for the Department of Health and the NHS on de-institutionalisation, community mental health services, violent mentally disordered offenders and assertive outreach teams. For the Department for Children Schools and Families (now Department of Education), he has researched the impact of Sure Start programmes, and the outcomes and costs of family support services and interagency training to safeguard children. He has also researched for the Department of Health and the Joseph Rowntree Foundation, the lives of disabled children and young people and their experiences of social care and health services.

John's other longstanding research is in the evaluation of interprofessional education and social work education. He is one of the leading international experts on these topics and is co-editor with Hilary Burgess of *The Outcomes of Social Work Education: developing evaluation methods* (Higher Education Academy, 2010) and of a forthcoming special issue of *Social Work Education* on outcomes research. John is currently leading a three-year longitudinal cohort study evaluating a national programme to support children's social workers in their first years in practice after qualification.

He is also currently working on the mental health of women migrant workers in China with Professor He Xuesong, Professor of Social Work at East China University of Science and Technology in Shanghai.

Professor Marion Bogo

Marion Bogo is Professor at the Factor-Inwentash Faculty of Social Work, University of Toronto, Canada. Her program of research and scholarship focuses on social work field education and clinical supervision, and the conceptualisation and assessment of professional competence. She has published over 100 journal articles and book chapters, and five books. Professor Bogo is a member of numerous journal editorial boards and was Associate Editor North America for *Social Work Education: The International Journal*. In 2013 she was awarded the Significant Lifetime Achievement in Social Work Education Award from the Council of Social Work Education, USA, in recognition of her contributions to social work education and to improving assessment of professional competence. In 2014 she was appointed as an Officer of the Order of Canada for her achievements in the field of social work as a scholar and teacher, and for advancing the practice in Canada and abroad.

Correspondence to: marion.bogo@utoronto.ca

Jane Paterson

Jane Paterson, MSW RSW is the director of interprofessional practice at the Centre for Addiction and Mental Health (CAMH) in Toronto. Her clinical work has involved working with people with co-occurring substance use and mental health problems and she has extensive experience in family treatment. In her current role, she has been involved in leading practice change initiatives and has established structures to support and mentor clinical staff. Her current work involves clinical policy development and implementation, student education and training, and promoting optimal care and learning through interprofessional education and collaboration. She has published in the areas of clinical supervision and electronic documentation. She is cross appointed to the Factor Inwentash Faculty of Social Work, University of Toronto and to Smith College School of Social Work, Northampton, Massachusetts.

Allyson Davys

Allyson Davys is an educator and a supervisor in private practice. Allyson has a long established interest and experience in interprofessional learning, working and supervision. Over the past 20 years she has run her own private supervision practice, was a senior lecturer at the University of Auckland teaching on the professional supervision programme and more recently for seven years was the centre director for the Centre for Health and Social Practice at the Waikato Institute of Technology. She has researched and published articles on professional supervision which have been published in local and international journals. With Liz Beddoe she co-authored a textbook on supervision *Best Practice in Professional Supervision: A Guide for the Helping Professions* (Jessica Kingsley Publishers, 2010).

Allyson is currently a PhD candidate in the School of Counselling, Human Services and Social Work at the University of Auckland.

Correspondence to: allyson.davys@gmail.com

Professor Liz Beddoe

Liz Beddoe is an Associate Professor in the School of Counselling, Human Services and Social Work at the University of Auckland in New Zealand. Liz's teaching and research interests include critical perspectives on social work education, professional supervision, and the media framing of social problems. Liz has published articles on supervision and professional issues in New Zealand and international journals. She has co-authored *Best Practice in Professional Supervision: A guide for the helping professions* (Jessica Kingsley Publishers, 2010) with Allyson Davys and *Mapping Knowledge for Social Work Practice: Critical intersections*, with Jane Maidment (2009, Cengage). She has co-edited *Promoting Health and Wellbeing in Social Work Education* (Routledge, 2013) with Beth Crisp and *Social Work Practice for Promoting Health and Wellbeing: Critical issues* with Jane Maidment (Routledge, 2014). *Supervision in Social Work: Contemporary issues*, an edited book, was published in March 2015 (Routledge).

Correspondence to: e.beddoe@auckland.ac.nz

Dr Tish Marrable

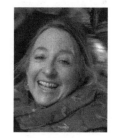

Tish Marrable is a lecturer in social work and social care at the University of Sussex. Recent research has focused on good supervision practices in adult integrated services, using a systems methodology to provide a holistic view of approaches. Other research includes work in interprofessional services for children and families, service access for adults with autistic spectrum conditions and research with carers into accessing services and interactions with social work. Her doctoral research, funded by the ESRC, explored the impact of emotion on the ways in which children and young people become identified and defined as having the need for extra help within children's services, and the ramifications for service provision. New work focuses on professional practice in the Rapid Response protocol when a child dies suddenly and unexpectedly in the home. Tish has a keen interest in social justice and how different approaches to this affect both policy and personal practice in social services. Before coming to academia she worked in a wide variety of areas including counselling, secondary schools, health and social care.

Sharon Lambley

Sharon Lambley is a lecturer in social work at the University of Sussex. She is a qualified and registered social worker and teacher, and has a master's in business administration. Her research interests lie in the interface between leadership, management and worker practices with service users, within shifting agency and policy contexts. Sharon is currently working with local agencies on evaluating the impact of learning, having developed a tool with agencies, managers, service users and teaching staff. Previous to this, she completed a research study on good and/or innovative supervision. Sharon has also completed research on workforce planning, workforce development, organisational development (including business development) and change. She has completed research on teaching and learning and the evaluation of learning. Sharon has worked collaboratively with researchers from other disciplines and other countries, and has carried out bespoke research for agencies, for example the NHS. Sharon has worked as a business development manager, social worker, manager, teaching fellow and researcher. She has a keen interest the role of service users in knowledge production, service design, delivery and evaluation. Her current work is focused on understanding supervision in situated contexts.

Jane Wonnacott

Jane Wonnacott is director of professional practice at In-Trac Training and Consultancy Ltd. She qualified as a social worker in 1979 and for the past 20 years has been working as an independent trainer and consultant. In this role she has worked with numerous statutory and voluntary organisations developing and delivering training as well as working on other projects including practice audits, policy development and serious case reviews. Jane has a long-standing interest in supervision and has developed and delivered supervision training courses both in the UK and abroad. She co-wrote, with Tony Morrison, the Children's Workforce Development Council's guide and training programme for the supervisors of social workers in the first three years of their professional development. Since Tony's death in 2010, In-Trac have continued to develop these training materials and from 2009–2014 trained over 10,000 supervisors working within health and social care. Jane is also author of *Mastering Social Work Supervision* (2012), published by Jessica Kingsley Publishers.

Dr Sonya Wallbank

Dr Sonya Wallbank is the founder and CEO of Fiduciam UK Ltd. As the original developer of the restorative programme of supervision in 2009, Sonya has maintained a strong belief that resilient staff are much more able to deliver their role effectively.

Sonya is a chartered psychologist by background and an associate fellow of the British Psychological Society (BPS). Sonya is also a registered member of the Health and Care Professional Council (HCPC) and chartered member of the Chartered Institute of Personnel Development (CIPD).

Sonya is the founder of Capellas Nurseries Group and has worked in the UK, USA and Australia training a range of staff to utilise her model within their work. Her most recent NHS position was Director of Children and Families. She has trained a range of staff in the NHS, Department of Health, local authorities, private organisations, hospices and charities. As a keen writer, Sonya has published in both professional journals and books and has a number of ongoing blogs.

Andy Bradley

In 2012 Andy Bradley was recognised by The Observer newspaper and NESTA as one of 'Britain's 50 Radicals' – his belief is that when we are vulnerable we should be met with consistent kindness and that we must 'elevate the status of care giving'. Andy created Frameworks 4 Change in 2004. Having spent part of his childhood living in a care home for people with dementia, Andy went on to give hands-on support to people with profound learning disabilities and older people and then to fill a range of leadership positions. Andy and the team at Frameworks 4 Change work hard every day to 'build a legacy of compassion in health and social care'. The habit building programmes that Andy now designs and facilitates with the team at Frameworks 4 Change are seeing dramatic results with continuous improvements to care and staff teams feeling valued and appreciated. Andy is currently working with the NHS, Local Authorities and a range of care provider organisations. Follow Andy and the work he does with many people up down the UK:

Twitter: @www.frameworks4c

Facebook.com/frameworks4change

Website: www.frameworks4change.co.uk

Rhiannon Barker

Rhiannon is head of business development at The Point of Care Foundation. Rhiannon is currently responsible for helping to identify, plan and test the development of new initiatives.

The foundation's mission is to keep patients' experience of care high on the agenda of policy makers and boards, and to work with managers and front-line staff to improve the experiences of both staff and patients. The foundation grew out of the work of the Point of Care programme at the King's Fund (2007-2013).

Rhiannon spent her early career in overseas development conducting evaluations of food aid distributions and then managing an oral history project across Sahelian Africa. Following that she worked as a research manager at the Health Education Authority and then became a freelance consultant specialising in qualitative health research, with broad experience across the voluntary and statutory sectors. She was a non-executive director at East Sussex Downs Primary Care Trust.

Dr Esther Flanagan

Esther is the Schwartz programme manager at The Point of Care Foundation. Her role is to help support staff to set up and sustain Schwartz Rounds, which 120 healthcare organisations have now committed to across the UK.

Esther qualified as a clinical psychologist at University College London and works with patients who have chronic pain conditions. She has a special interest in the use of technology for delivery of psychological therapies and training. Esther also worked at the National Collaborating Centre for Mental Health, where she was project managing several guidelines on mental health issues.

Jeremy Winter

Jeremy Winter was born in 1959 in Shropshire, and graduated with a science degree from Southampton University, but then changed direction, achieving a CQSW after a two-year postgraduate course in social work at Lancaster University in 1990. Having previously worked in supporting adults with learning disabilities in the community in Preston, Jeremy joined a multidisciplinary team working with adults with learning disabilities and challenging behaviour in East Lancashire. He worked in a number of adult learning disability teams, moving into management in due course. Jeremy currently works for Lancashire County Council as an advanced practitioner, seeking to support and encourage social workers to be the best practitioners they can be in a fast changing social care environment.

Correspondence to: jeremy.winter@lancashire.gov.uk

Kevin Brett

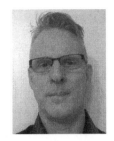

After several years in the military, Kevin Brett trained as a registered general nurse before undertaking further training as a paediatric nurse, specialising in intensive care of sick and premature infants. He worked for several years in the Middle East and Australia, including providing heath care and support to aboriginal communities in the Australian outback.

Following time working in major teaching hospitals in Central London he developed a career within community health care, working as an advanced practitioner before moving into operational management.

Kevin's current managerial role is the first where he has responsibility for health and social care teams. They provide support for people within the locality to avoid unnecessary hospital admissions and to facilitate timely discharges.

Maryam Zonouzi

Maryam Zonouzi is a social entrepreneur, academic, disability activist and business and technology innovator. She worked in the voluntary sector before moving into social enterprise as a way of accelerating change for individuals with care and support needs.

Maryam is the co-author of *Personalisation and Social Work and Community Health Nursing* (5th Edition) where she wrote extensively on co-production and patient and public engagement. Her academic and research interests include exploring how to disrupt professional practice to improve the lives of service users and professionals alike. Maryam is currently a researcher at the Tilda Goldberg Centre researching the impact of reclaiming social work.

Paul David Spencer Ross

Paul David Spencer Ross is a senior information specialist within the Social Care Institute for Excellence (SCIE) which hosts the NICE Collaborating Centre for Social Care. Paul is a chartered member of the Chartered Institute of Library and Information Professionals and has worked on a variety of topics across the social care sector. He specialises in community facilitation and knowledge growth through information and resource forums for minority and unheard groups, along with practical training in searching skills for social care research evidence.

Lisa Smith

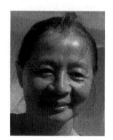

Lisa Smith, research and development manager, joined Research in Practice for Adults (RiPfA) in July 2013, following over four years of working in a commissioning role for Torbay Council. Prior to this she worked as a practice based commissioning advisor, working with GP consortia. Lisa is experienced in service redesign and development, having worked as the lead for the Bristol Drug Strategy Team in the implementation of Models of Care. Lisa has a background in research having worked for a number of years at the University of Bath in the Mental Health Research and Development Unit as both a researcher and a research governance facilitator.

Meiling Kam

Meiling Kam is a registered social worker and a practice development manager at the Social Care Institute for Excellence. She produced and co-wrote a suite of resources on effective supervision in social work and social care, a guide on care home residents' access to GP services and a number of other resources available online. She also writes children's books.

Foreword

Lyn Romeo, Chief Social Worker, Department of Health

When I look back over my social work career, I know that what made the real difference to improving my practice and ensuring the people I worked with achieved the best possible outcomes, was the quality of supervision I was afforded.

Practice supervision has not had enough attention in mainstream social work and social care practice with adults. In social work with disabled and older people with social care needs, the recent history of process-led approaches to assessment, care management, eligibility decisions and resource allocation has put the emphasis on managerial supervision. Residential and home care services for adults lack a strong tradition of practice supervision: its availability is patchy, its quality variable.

Reflective practice supervision in work with adults is more important than ever in ensuring that attention is paid to the actual social work, the relationships and personal interactions that take place between the social worker and the person and family with whom they are working. This is essential in rebalancing the managerial supervision approaches which are fairly well embedded.

With the increasing integration of health and social care, social workers in multiprofessional teams and services need access to the right level of skilled social work practice supervision. This should normally come from a social-work-trained supervisor, to ensure that as a profession we have a relentless focus on improving social work practice. It will also be key in positioning social work as a vital part of effective integrated health and social care services.

Putting the service user at the centre involves a challenging culture shift for many practitioners, especially where the person's wishes and the outcomes they want for themselves do not fit with the agenda of the organisation and its performance targets. We must listen to and learn from the people we work with, their families and carers, if we are to improve and inform social work and social care practice for the future. Reflective supervision helps to tease out and consolidate that learning.

We must also continue our efforts to enhance the evidence base for the effectiveness of social work and social care interventions, and the outcomes they enable people and carers to achieve. Every day, social workers in adult social care are working with legal complexities, risk, conflict and uncertainty, and having to make well-evidenced professional judgements to support what is in the best interests of individuals and their carers. High quality supervision is important in supporting social workers to think through the issues, dilemmas and best practice approaches to different individuals' situations. It also enables a robust response to ongoing challenges regarding the place of social care and social work in the developing health and social care landscape.

Good practice supervision also supports the adoption of more explicit theoretical models of practice and provision, and helps to ensure meaningful engagement with individuals and their families. We have opportunities to develop innovative approaches to practice supervision and improvements that remain person-centred, and involve face-to-face or written feedback from people with first-hand experience of social work involvement.

Strong, effective, practice leadership in social work with adults is a key driver in improving social work practice, promoting well-being and implementing the personalised community-focused approaches set out in the Care Act (2014). Good practice will come from leaders ensuring workloads are manageable, prioritising training and development and providing supportive, challenging supervision that attends to the quality of social work practice.

I welcome this book and the attention it gives to different models of supervision in the variety of settings, some of them interprofessional, within which social workers' practice and social care is delivered. It is great that there is a strong focus on outcomes for service users, a chapter that looks at involving service users in supervision and another looking at emerging models of supervision that are service user led. Recognising and developing compassionate care is a recurrent theme. If we can get this right, then we really can deliver excellent social work and social care practice for those with whom we are privileged to work.

Editorial

Interprofessional supervision

Dr Lisa Bostock

It has been a privilege to curate this book and to bring together a unique collection of perspectives from within the UK and overseas on interprofessional supervision in services to adults. I have always supervised staff from different disciplinary backgrounds to my own and enjoyed the intellectual frisson of being introduced to new ways of thinking about research and practice development. Indeed, my current staff team includes service user researchers, social workers, psychologists, criminologists and a former financial journalist turned children's participation expert! I also know from a personal perspective the challenges of working together effectively, and that interprofessional supervision works best when built on a foundation of positive team relationships and mutual respect for professional differences.

This book is about what makes interprofessional supervision a success. There has been an international shift toward this form of supervision, driven by a broad consensus that multidisciplinary teams produce better outcomes for service users, combined with a cost saving agenda in which integrated working is seen as the key to increased financial efficiency. Yet it is an area where practice is ahead of the research; few studies have investigated how best to deliver effective supervision across disciplinary boundaries. What evidence exists tends to focus on services for children; there is a dearth of information on supervising staff working in adult services.

This book represents an opportunity to address this gap in the evidence base and offers approaches to staff supervision from across a variety of different professional perspectives and practice settings. It draws together a unique blend of researchers, practitioners and service users who identify both the opportunities and challenges of interprofessional supervision, as well as explore what works best in which context, for whom and why. It is concerned with the outcomes of this type of supervision for organisations, workers and ultimately service users. Contributions cover social work, healthcare (including hospitals, nursing and midwifery), residential care, community learning disability, mental health and addiction services as well as supervision of personal assistants. The book looks beyond the UK and presents international evidence of the incidence and experience of interprofessional supervision with contributions from Canada and New Zealand.

The book is divided into three sections. The first part provides an international overview of key research on interprofessional supervision. It includes an update on recent UK policy and practice developments as well as a discussion of service user involvement in staff supervision. The second section looks at innovative approaches to supervision and explores models developed in a variety of practice domains. The third section provides personal accounts of peoples' experiences of this type of supervision, and includes contributions from service managers and service users. It concludes with reflections on the core themes of the book, making suggestions for where next for research on supervision in adult services. The research digest section in this volume has been compiled by Paul David Spencer Ross from the Social Care Institute for Excellence (SCIE). There is also a short final section of some hand-picked useful tools and resources.

Supervision, and the role of the supervisor, have become more crucial than ever. The worlds of social care and health care are undergoing rapid change. Traditional roles and boundaries are less well defined, and new service models are emerging. Some of the changes are the result of political intent and policy decisions, including a commitment to integrated working for the benefit of people with multiple conditions and multiple health and care needs. Some reflect the continuing growth in knowledge from research and development, from the experience and feedback of people using services, and from technological advances. Some changes are the consequence of competing pressures; of growing demand, rising expectations, increasing complexity, shifting priorities, tighter regulation and constrained resources.

Taken together, the changes have created a context for practice and service provision where the emphasis is on fostering independence and self-help, preventing health deterioration, managing risk and safeguarding from abuse, maximising choice, encouraging flexibility and innovation, and making efficient use of all the available resources. In this sometimes bewildering environment, the supervisor is key to supporting and guiding practitioners by keeping their attention on the needs of individuals and families, clarifying the outcomes they are seeking to achieve, sharing the assessment and management of risk, forestalling problems and encouraging reflective learning, overseeing their professional development and staying alert to their personal situations. Staff cannot provide quality support and care for others unless they themselves feel well-supported and looked after.

Part I:

Interprofessional supervision: Policy context and messages from research

Introduction to Part I

Part I provides busy practitioners with an accessible account of latest thinking, research and policy debates on supervision. Authors in this section of the book focus specifically on what we mean by effective supervision within integrated and multidisciplinary settings, how is it conducted and how do we know that it makes a difference. They pose the question 'does it matter if supervisors are from a different professional background to supervisees, if the key ingredients are the same?'

Chapter 1 looks at drivers for change within the UK policy and practice context. This chapter is written by Don Brand, social care consultant, policy analyst and former deputy chief inspector at the Social Services Inspectorate. He discusses the implications of changing demographics, public spending cuts and recent legislative changes for staff supervision in adult services. This means that supervisors of health and social care professionals are constantly required to adapt and diversify as people's needs, policies, provision and practice change.

Chapter 2 is co-authored by social work researchers, Caroline Webb, Lisa Bostock and leading social work academic John Carpenter. This is based on an international, systematic review of the research literature on effective supervision in social work and social care. This chapter reports on the paucity of evidence on the impact of supervision in services for adults. It notes that while the evidence that exists has largely been conducted in integrated services, only two studies explore in any detail how supervision operates within a multidisciplinary setting.

One of these studies is the focus of Chapter 3. Award-winning social work academic Marion Bogo and Jane Paterson, director of interprofessional practice and researcher, present findings from their study of interprofessional supervision at Canada's largest mental health and addiction hospital, the newly amalgamated Centre for Addiction and Mental Health (CAMH) in Toronto. With some exceptions, practitioners from across professions identified three inter-related components of quality supervision: structure, process, and content. When present, supervision was valued by workers regardless of the supervisor's professional discipline. Nevertheless, authors note the importance of organisational context to the success of supervision.

Chapter 4 reviews the wider literature on the incidence and experience of interprofessional supervision within specific professions. New Zealand based social work academics Allyson Davys and Liz Beddoe identify an international shift toward this form of supervision reflecting trends toward multidisciplinary working. The studies they identify largely report worker satisfaction with this type of supervision, although challenges as well as benefits are explored.

Finally, Chapter 5 looks specifically at the role of an overlooked but key stakeholder in supervision; the service user. Social work academics Tish Marrable and Sharon Lambley ask us to consider service user involvement in supervision, drawing on unique research with service users, frontline workers and their managers working in integrated settings.

Chapter 1

Supervision across interprofessional boundaries in services aimed at adults: The policy context for supervision

Don Brand MBE

Introduction

The policy context for supervision of practice and provision is dominated by demographics, whether in adult social care, health care or housing. All services face the challenge of meeting the needs of steeply rising numbers of older people and making proper provision for more severely disabled and sensory-impaired people of working age. All except the NHS are subject to substantial cuts in public funding.

The section of the population aged 85 and over is the fastest growing age group in the UK. Their numbers have risen by nearly 680,000 in 25 years, reaching 1.3 million in 2007. ONS projections suggest that by 2033, the number will reach 3.3 million. These trends will increase significantly the demand for social support and care, health care and treatment, housing, income support and benefits.

The growing population of much older people means a direct increase in the numbers with conditions like diabetes or dementia, where prevalence increases with age. Older people with multiple long-term conditions will increase in number from just over two million in 2013 to 2.9 million by 2018. Many people have complex combinations of physical, intellectual and mental health impairments. Depression is seven times more common in people with two or more chronic physical conditions than in those with none. Yet NHS services and professional structures generally reflect individual clinical conditions, and it is not always easy to ensure integrated NHS responses to people with multiple health needs.

There is growing understanding of the risks to disabled and older people of neglect, exploitation, harassment and abuse. It is not clear whether increases in referrals reflect greater incidence of mistreatment, or increased awareness of these risks among professionals. Exposure of gross maltreatment of learning disabled people by staff at Winterbourne View Hospital has highlighted the particular problems of people whose behaviour others find challenging. Police use of 'hate crime' definitions has led to greater focus on harassment and abuse of disabled people and those with learning difficulties, and ways of tackling and preventing these problems.

The past five years have seen significant policy and financial changes across all public services. Much of the change has been driven by strong downward pressures on public spending levels in the name of deficit-reduction. There is broad political consensus in favour of the concept of health and social care integration. Some of the measures government expect to secure savings – increased competition, talking up prevention/diversion, emphasising self-help, strengthening community support networks – rest more on ideological preferences and optimistic assumptions than robust evidence. This means that staff supervision across professional boundaries takes place in an ever-changing and highly pressurised policy and practice context.

Purposes of supervision

The term 'supervision' carries a variety of connotations in different professional and organisational settings. For some professionals, supervision is associated with training and perhaps an initial period in practice. After that, when the individual has achieved independent professional status, there would be no expectation of supervision continuing. In other professions, including social work, supervision from a more experienced colleague is accepted as an integral part of continuing professional development and helps to challenge assumptions, reflect on practice and decisions etc. It is also a vital means of protecting the well-being of both the people receiving services and the practitioner, and is an essential element of the employer's duty of care.

The main purposes of social care and health care supervision include:

→ improving well-being and outcomes for service users and carers

→ maintaining and enhancing quality and practice standards, informed by the best evidence from research, user expertise and practice knowledge

→ safeguarding people using services, the worker and colleagues, and the public

→ managing accountability and compliance with statutory requirements and guidance, plus employer's policies, procedures and financial controls

→ developmental and pastoral support to practitioners and providers.

Common policy context for adult health, social care and related services

Across the four UK administrations – England, Wales, Scotland and Northern Ireland – there are a number of common themes concerning the context for interprofessional supervision. There is consensus that service provision and practice should be personalised and person-centred, designed to enable people needing care and support to enjoy maximum independence, choice and control. Policy and guidance require maximum user participation in the design, planning, development, delivery, review and regulation of services.

There is general agreement that the provision of support should be based on an all-round assessment of a person's needs, strengths, aspirations and preferences. Such an assessment can be co-produced by the person and the professionals working together on an equal footing, with scope for self-assessment and recognising the benefits of self-directed support. People and their carers should have ready access to the information and advice that enables them to stay independent and in control.

Policy in all parts of the UK emphasises helping people to maintain their capacity, to avoid and recover from breakdown, and through timely access to re-ablement services, to restore lost capability. It also promotes increasing investment to support carers to sustain their contribution to meeting the care and support needs of relatives and friends, by ensuring they have realistic options to engage in education or employment and helping them manage other caring responsibilities within the family.

Within different central and local government structures, all four administrations are seeking to create flexible models for co-ordinating social care, health, housing, welfare, transport, employment, education and training facilities. A central challenge is to build innovative, co-ordinated, community-oriented and complementary health and care provision and support networks.

As we have seen, social care and the NHS are dealing with growing numbers of people with multiple and complex conditions and rising expectations of control, choice and independence, living in community settings and requiring robust, skilled and specialist treatment, care and support. These trends present far-reaching implications for management and leadership development, education and training of the workforce, and more dynamic systems of staff and service regulation.

Legislative and policy context – England

The position before 2015

The legislative framework in England for adult social care accumulated piecemeal over 65 years, between the National Assistance Act (1948) and the Health and Social Care Act (2012). The 1948 act replaced the Poor Law (1834), but some of the values and assumptions of the Poor Law carried over into the new 1948 act and its implementation. The National Health Service was designed from the outset as a universal service, available to all, free at the point of need, nationally administered, its costs pooled and met from taxation; whereas services under the 1948 act were restricted to those found to be in need of care and attention not otherwise available to them, administered by local authorities and subject to a means test. This division largely remains, and obstructs joint working.

The stream of policy documents issued and statutes passed between 1948 and 2012 greatly extended the range and purposes of adult social care. Legislation recognised new types of need, further groups who qualified for help and different ways for authorities to respond. Key statutes included the Chronically Sick and Disabled Persons Act (1970), the Mental Health Act (1983), the NHS and Community Care Act (1990), The Carers (Recognition and Services) Act (1995), the Community Care (Direct Payments) Act (1996), the Mental Capacity Acts (2005, 2007), the Safeguarding Vulnerable Groups Act (2006), and the Equality Acts (2006, 2010).

Each of these acts reflected the values, language and assumptions of its own times. Governments had long recognised the need to consolidate and modernise adult social care law, just as the law relating to children and families has been brought together in the Children Act (1989). In 2008, the Law Commission was asked to review adult social care law in England and Wales and make recommendations to replace it with a single modern statute. The Commission issued a final report in May 2011, with recommendations for the structure and contents of separate bills for England and Wales. The bills consolidated much existing legislation, but excluded the Mental Health Act and Mental Capacity Acts.

The Care Act (2014)

In July 2012 the Government issued a response to the Law Commission's report and a draft Care and Support Bill for England. The Law Commissioner Frances Patterson, who had led the project, commented:

'The government has accepted our thinking that the individual should be at the heart of the new statute, and that the guiding principle of care and support is to promote the well-being of the individual and focus on their needs and aspirations, rather than those of the local authority or service provider. The government has also accepted our reforms for carers.'

The government's draft bill was subject to further public consultation and to pre-legislative scrutiny by a Parliamentary Committee. The Care Bill was introduced in the House of Lords in May 2013, was debated and amended there and transferred as amended to the House of Commons in October 2013. It received Royal Assent as the Care Act in May 2014.

The well-being principle

Clause 1 of the Care Act defines the over-arching principle of the act as *'promoting the well-being of the individual.'* This is the touchstone for all local authority functions under the act; including prevention, safeguarding, need and eligibility assessments, development and review of individual care and support plans, plus ensuring a diverse range of high-quality provision. As these functions increasingly take place in integrated settings, supervisors will have to apply the well-being principle to interprofessional working.

Clause 1 goes on to define the different domains of people's lives in which the well-being principle applies and to specify how to engage people in decisions that affect them. This effectively enshrines in statute, for the first time, the key elements of personalisation and independent living. It also encourages a holistic understanding of the key aspects of people's lives and the scope for flexible, creative and innovative responses to needs.

Domains of well-being (Care Act (2014) Clause 1(2))

(a) personal dignity (including treatment of the individual with respect)

(b) physical and mental health and emotional well-being

(c) protection from abuse and neglect

(d) control by the individual over day-to-day life....

(e) participation in work, education, training or recreation

(f) social and economic well-being

(g) domestic, family and personal relationships

(h) suitability of living accommodation

(i) the individual's contribution to society.

(Care Act (2014) © Crown Copyright 2015)

Principles of personalisation (Care Act Clause 1(3))

(a) starting with the person's view of what's best for them

(b) taking full account of their views, wishes, feelings and beliefs

(c) preventing, delaying or reducing care and support needs

(d) taking all the person's circumstances into account in decisions

(e) providing the person with information and support to participate in decisions

(f) achieving a balance between the person's well-being and that of any carers

(g) ensuring people are protected from abuse and neglect

(h) finding the route that least restricts the person's rights and freedoms.

(Care Act (2014) © Crown Copyright 2015)

Needs assessment and care and support planning

The Care Act introduces a new needs assessment framework. This obliges a local authority to carry out a needs assessment where it appears to them that an adult may have needs for care and support, and apply national eligibility criteria to judge who qualifies for support and care. If the person's needs meet the eligibility criteria, the local authority must work with the person, carers and relatives to prepare and implement a care and support plan.

Under the act, carers who appear to have needs for support also qualify for a needs assessment, and a decision on whether their needs meet the eligibility criteria for support. If so, the act strengthens their right to support. The needs may be met either by providing support to the carer, or by increasing provision of care and support to the person for whom they care. A support plan will set out the details.

Funding care and support

In the person's care and support plan, the local authority will set out its assessment of the costs of meeting their eligible needs and the level of charges the person is expected to meet. The authority's net contribution may then take the form of direct service provision; a care budget, allocated by or on behalf of the individual, giving more control of how, when and by whom care and support is provided; or a direct payment to buy in and manage the care and support they choose. Those with health as well as care needs may be able to integrate personal budgets for health and social care and create flexible personalised health and care packages.

Transition from children's to adults' services

The Care Act contains provisions relating to two other topics with multi-agency and multidisciplinary dimensions. The first is supporting disabled young people and their families through the transition from children's to adults' services. Parents had long expressed serious concerns about the arbitrary reductions in quantity and quality of support services their children experienced, simply because they turned 18 years old. The transfer to adult services frequently came as a shock, with a greatly reduced level and range of resources available to them, and an expectation that they would simply accept narrowed horizons.

The Care Act, taken in conjunction with the Children and Families Act (2014), provides for more active and proactive co-ordination between children's and adults' services in supporting disabled young people and families through the transition process. The Children and Families Act establishes new procedures to ensure disabled young people's education, health and care needs are assessed and met within a single integrated framework, leading to the preparation of an individual Health, Education and Care Plan (EHC) which can continue until the young person reaches twenty-five years old. Under the Care Act, a local authority must assess the care and support needs of a young person during the year before they turn 18. The purpose is to determine what their care and support needs may be after they turn 18 and to ensure a care and support plan is in place to meet their eligible needs and the support needs of their carers.

Adult safeguarding

The other key area for joint working is local arrangements for adult safeguarding. Under the act, the local authority must identify each person with needs for care and support who is experiencing, or is at risk of, abuse or neglect, and is unable to protect himself or herself against them. For each person at risk, it must decide whether any action is required and if so, what action is needed and who should take it.

The local authority is also responsible for convening the local inter-agency Safeguarding Adult Board (SAB). The board brings together the agencies with responsibilities in relation to adult safeguarding, and conducts Safeguarding Adult Reviews (SARs). A review is required if an adult experiencing abuse or neglect dies as a result (or survives but is known to have suffered severe abuse or neglect) and there is reasonable cause for concern about how the agencies worked together to safeguard the adult.

Health and social care integration

More integrated working between adult social care and the NHS is a policy principle to which governments have subscribed for decades. As well as regular exhortations to collaborate, and integrating service regulation through the Care Quality Commission, ministers have tried a range of schemes and initiatives to promote joint working. Over the years, these have included:

→ earmarked joint finance allocations

→ protocols for joint assessment by health and social care staff

→ provisions for pooled health and care budgets

→ local Joint Strategic Needs Assessments

→ local Joint Health and Wellbeing Boards and Health and Wellbeing Strategies

→ the national Better Care Fund, allocated to local authorities and their health partners to implement the Care Act, reduce emergency admissions, and deliver specified service improvements including seven-day-working.

The Health and Social Care Act (2012) and the Care Act (2014) contain complementary provisions to secure commitments to integrated working by the NHS and local authorities, the latter with responsibilities for adult social care, public health, housing, planning, children and family services, and education. The Department of Health's fact sheet about the Health and Social Care Act states:

'Improving quality of care is at the heart of the Health and Social Care Act 2012. One key means to achieve this is to ensure care is integrated around the needs of patients. Typically the NHS has not managed handovers well between different parts of the NHS, or with social care. As such, the Act seeks to encourage and enable more integration between services.' (Department of Health, 2012)

Section 3 of the Care Act expects the local authority to play its part in ensuring the integration of care and support provision with health and health-related provision, in order to promote adult and carer well-being, contribute to prevention, and improve quality of care and support. Interestingly it says, *'for the purposes of this section, the provision of housing is a health-related provision.'*

During the passage of the 2012 Bill, the Government asked the NHS Future Forum to consult widely on specific aspects of the NHS reforms. One of the Forum's stakeholder groups was commissioned to report on integration. They said:

'Integration should be defined around the patient, not the system ....'

'Health and wellbeing boards should drive local integration – through a whole-population, strategic approach that addresses local priorities.' (NHS Future Forum, 2012)

Most critically:

'The Forum heard a consistent message from patients, service users, carers, clinicians and managers that integration is only valuable insofar as it improves experience and outcomes for the individual. It is not a virtue in its own right, but one important aspect of the quality of care.' (NHS Future Forum, 2012)

The future of interprofessional supervision

Following the 2015 election, the Government has established a series of inter-ministerial implementation task forces to resolve complex long-term policy issues. The Health and Social Care Implementation Taskforce has the remit *'to deliver an integrated health and social care system.'*

Ministers have renounced further organisational re-structuring. If this self-denying ordinance holds, more organic, flexible and innovative forms of joint working and integrated provision can be expected to emerge. Interprofessional working across the NHS and social care will expand further, adapting and diversifying as needs, policies, provision and practice change.

This will necessitate skilled and knowledgeable interprofessional supervision. Supervisors will need to understand the values and expertise of different professions, know how to promote co-operation and manage conflict, and ensure that the well-being of the individual is the priority of all.

References

Department of Health (2012) *Improving Integration of Services: The Health and Social Care Act 2012* [online]. Available at: https://www.gov.uk/government/uploads/system/uploads/attachment_data/file/138268/C3.-Factsheet-Promoting-better-integration-of-health-and-care-services-270412.pdf (accessed November 2015)

NHS Future Forum (2012) *Summary Report: Second Phase* [online]. Available at: http://webarchive.nationalarchives.gov.uk/20130805112926/https://www.gov.uk/government/uploads/system/uploads/attachment_data/file/216422/dh_132085.pdf (accessed November 2015)

Chapter 2

Effective supervision in social work and social care: Findings from a systematic review of research in services to adults (2000-2012)

Caroline Webb, Dr Lisa Bostock and Professor John Carpenter

Introduction and general overview of the studies

What do we mean by 'supervision'?

Although supervision has been described as *'an integral element of social work practice not an add-on'* (DCSF, 2009) there is no universal definition of what 'supervision' actually is, and it may mean different things to different professionals. Within the social work profession, the British Association of Social Workers suggests that the *'prime purpose'* of supervision is to support workers to provide good quality services and *'maximise their effectiveness'* (BASW & CSW, 2011).

There are several key functions of supervision that are consistently identified within the literature: administrative/case management, reflecting on and learning from practice, personal support, mediation (the supervisor acts as a 'bridge' between worker and organisation) and professional development (Carpenter *et al*, 2012).

Why is supervision important?

'The overall aim of professional supervision should be to provide the best possible support to service users in accordance with the organisation's responsibilities and accountable professional standards.' (Carpenter *et al*, 2012)

Organisations can hope to achieve this by ensuring that their staff are skilled, knowledgeable, clear about their job roles, and offered practical assistance from a supervisor in the form of job-related advice and emotional support. Organisations also have a duty of care to their staff, and providing good quality supervision will help to ensure workers' well-being and job satisfaction, and may mean they are more likely to remain in their jobs.

Supervision in practice: some cautionary remarks

Although clearly important, the delivery of high quality supervision in practice may not be an easy task. Organisations are experiencing increasing pressure on resources and accountability, and worker's support and development needs may get replaced by performance measurement and management oversight. The Social Work Task Force (DCSF, 2009) reported that social workers in England were receiving variable access to supervision, which was largely process-driven and focused on case management.

Although policy makers, educators and practitioners generally assume that supervision is a 'good thing', there is in fact a distinct lack of research evidence in relation to social work supervision. Indeed the evidence base has been described as *'surprisingly weak'*, and this makes it very difficult for organisations to apply evidence-based supervisory processes (Carpenter *et al*, 2013).

Concerns have also been raised in the UK about the supervision of social workers working in integrated and multi-disciplinary teams, as they may not always be supervised by fellow social workers (Cameron *et al*, 2012). The lack of research evidence on supervision makes it difficult to assess the impact on staff. As Carpenter *et al* (2012) ask: are the key supervisory ingredients the same, or are social work values and working practices unique to the discipline and therefore integral to the professional practice and development of practitioners?

Aim of this chapter

This chapter offers a summary of the research evidence on the value of supervision within adult social care. It provides an overview of the data derived from an international systematic review into effective supervision in social work and social care commissioned by the Social Care Institute for Excellence (SCIE) (Carpenter et al, 2012). This review explored outcomes for services to children and families as well as adult social care. While the focus is on social work and social care, some of the research reviewed includes workers from other professions such as nursing and psychology. The chapter will also examine the evidence on different models of supervision and the outcomes for workers, organisations, service users and carers as well as providing a focus on the evidence relating to supervision in integrated, multiprofessional teams. It concludes by discussing the potential implications for stakeholders along with suggestions for future research.

What does the research show?

Overview of the studies

This chapter draws on findings from 14 of the studies cited within the SCIE research briefing which focused on supervision within an adult context (the remaining studies concerned supervision in social work or social care within a children and families/child welfare setting) (see the Appendix for details of all the studies). Nine of the studies originated from the US (Allen et al, 2004; Bowers & Jacobson, 2002; Brannon et al, 2007; Cole et al, 2004; DeLoach & Monroe, 2004; Egan & Kadushin, 2004; Kim & Lee, 2009; Lee & del Carmen Montiel, 2011; Simons & Jankowski, 2007), one stemmed from Australia (Kavanagh et al, 2003), two from Canada (Bogo et al, 2011a; 2011b), one from Israel (Ben-Porat & Itzhaky, 2011) and just one study from the UK (Fleming & Taylor, 2007).

Most of the studies (nine) collected quantitative survey data using a cross-sectional design (or in other words they collected numerical data at a single point in time), three of the studies reported on qualitative data (such as that deriving from interviews or focus groups with staff) while two adopted a mixed-methods approach using both quantitative and qualitative data (see Appendix). This means that most studies only reported on correlational evidence in which supervision featured as one factor among many that were associated with outcomes, such as workers' job satisfaction, stress or intention to leave.

Models of supervision

Manthorpe et al (2013) suggest that models of supervision are essentially dialectical or opposing in their approach: they are either 'introspective' (a therapeutic model) or 'instrumental' (a tool for the exercise of power and authority). An instrumental model of supervision primarily consists of administrative/case management functions designed to assess the performance of the employee in line with the organisation's duties and responsibilities. This contrasts with 'introspective' models of supervision which are often group-based and focus on the reflective or clinical functions, although reflective supervision can also occur outside of a group setting. For example an external supervisor may provide this while a workplace supervisor focuses on administrative needs, for example as occurs in Sweden (Bradley & Höjer, 2009).

Within the 14 studies reviewed, few details are offered about the exact nature of the supervision being provided. It appears that the most common supervisory approach uses an 'instrumental' model, where supervision is delivered via a one-to-one meeting with a supervisor which is presumably the worker's line manager, although this isn't often stated. No studies attempted to evaluate the outcomes of a supervisory intervention or model, nor is any specific data provided in relation to models of group supervision.

Supervision in multidisciplinary settings and interprofessional practice

Perhaps surprisingly, while 10 of the 14 studies were completed in interprofessional contexts, only the two qualitative studies by Bogo et al (2011a; 2011b) explore in any detail how supervision operates within an integrated setting. Conducted in Canada, these studies examine workers' views on the supervision arrangements following the amalgamation of two mental health and two addiction services. As a consequence of restructuring, some practitioners no longer received supervision from supervisors of the same professional background.

As reported by Bogo and Paterson in chapter 3 of this volume, workers described mixed reactions to the receipt of interprofessional supervision. Some staff reported that they missed having that connection to their own professional discipline and being able to 'talk in their own language.' They also now felt that supervision ignored clinical issues and focused solely on performance management. Tensions were also evident in relation to upholding the social work values of being non-judgemental and promoting empowerment, while maintaining a focus on client/public safety.

However, other practitioners were more positive and valued supervisors who attempted to understand the frameworks of their supervisee's profession. It was noted that participants perceived 'safety' and 'trust' to be more important than whether the supervisor was from the same profession. The key elements of valued supervisors were their clinical expertise and ability to provide new and relevant practice knowledge, while promoting learning in a respectful and safe way; almost all participants agreed these were more important than their professional affiliation.

Staff also reported that the new interprofessional teams were a valuable source of support, offering spontaneous and informal feedback in the face of critical and emotionally provocative experiences. Interestingly, these views did not appear to be related to their perceptions of their supervisor. This suggests that a worker's relationships with their colleagues and their relationship with their supervisor are separate constructs. However in cases where participants were the only member of their profession on the team, they did still value the chance to meet with others from their own occupation, perhaps as interprofessional supervision may not include profession-specific work.

Supervision and cost effectiveness

No studies included an economic evaluation of supervision. Economic evaluations identify, measure and compare the costs and outcomes of alternative interventions. In the area of supervision, this might include comparing the costs and outcomes of individual vs. group supervision, or supervision by a supervisor of the same profession compared with interprofessional supervision, for example. This is a significant gap in the evidence base given that staff retention is associated with good quality supervision, while high levels of turnover are linked to increased organisational costs, reduced effectiveness, and poorer outcomes for service users (Webb & Carpenter, 2012). This lack of research evidence means that we cannot say which type of supervision works best for whom, and in which context.

Supervision and outcomes for workers

The fields of social work and social care are widely acknowledged to place particular demands on staff, and it is an employer's responsibility to ensure that good quality supervision is provided as part of their duty of care to their workforce. The importance of supervision to outcomes for workers is a recurring theme in the literature with 13 of the 14 studies reviewed focusing on the links between supervision and worker outcomes. There is one exception – Bowers and Jacobson (2002) considered organisational outcomes only.

Positive outcomes for workers include:

→ increased job satisfaction

→ organisational commitment and intention to stay

→ social and emotional well-being.

Detrimental outcomes include:

→ intention to leave

→ stress

→ burnout

→ secondary traumatisation.

Beginning with beneficial outcomes, nine studies considered links between supervision and workers' job satisfaction (Allen *et al*, 2004; Bogo *et al*, 2011a; 2011b; Cole *et al*, 2004; DeLoach & Monroe, 2004; Egan & Kadushin, 2004; Kavanagh *et al*, 2003; Lee & del Carmen Montiel, 2011; Simons & Jankowski, 2007), six of which were conducted in in-professional contexts (see Appendix). The concept of job satisfaction is typically comprised of three key themes which these studies explored – 1) structure, focus and frequency of supervision 2) task assistance and 3) support to access resources for service users.

Job satisfaction: frequency of supervision

In general, greater frequency of supervision is associated with higher levels of satisfaction, with some studies reporting a minimum of two hours per week as a prerequisite to job satisfaction and retention (Carpenter *et al*, 2012). Bogo *et al*'s (2011a; 2011b) studies of clinical supervision found that regardless of whether respondents shared the same professional background, job satisfaction and professional development were related to the following key components of supervision: that it was regular, that it was provided by those with expert knowledge and clinical intervention skills for the specific client population, that it was able to teach new effective treatment methods, and that there was reciprocity and active involvement from supervisees.

Job satisfaction: task assistance

Task assistance involves a supervisor's tangible, work-related advice and instruction to a supervisee, and focuses on training, skills and solutions for practice (Mor Barak *et al*, 2009). It is related to positive outcomes for workers by supporting them to think through tasks and perform more effectively. In Ben-Porat and Itzhaky's (2011) study of therapists working with survivors

of domestic abuse in Israel, task assistance was of particular importance to workers in terms of role clarity – supporting them with perceived role competence and with task knowledge and problem-solving. Cole *et al* (2004) reported in their US study of social workers that perceived quality of supervision was predictive of job satisfaction in a multiple regression analysis. The mentoring function of supervision in relation to practitioners' job satisfaction, including assigning workers challenging tasks, is also highlighted in a small scale study of mental health workers and supervisors in the US (Lee & del Carmen Montiel, 2011).

Job satisfaction: access to resources

The impact of accessing support for service users is explored in a study of home health social workers in the US (Egan & Kadushin, 2004). They found that helpfulness of 'administrators' (i.e. budget-holders) in resolving difficulties between patient access to services and financial priorities, contributed significantly to greater job satisfaction. Egan and Kadushin conclude that in this cost-conscious context, 'administrative' supervision (whereby supervisors provide support so that staff can access resources to meet patient need and thus resolve their own ethical conflicts or uneasiness about not being able to offer services) is more important than 'emotional' supervision focused on professional development and mentoring. This demonstrates the context-dependant nature of supervision and its association with workers' job satisfaction.

Organisational commitment

Supervision is also associated with other beneficial worker outcomes such as increased organisational commitment and workers' overall social and emotional well-being. Allen *et al* (2004) looked at social work and human services workers in the US, and found that supervision was significantly linked to workers' organisational commitment. This suggests that the degree to which employees feel supported by their supervisor contributes to their overall appraisal of how the organisation values and cares about them.

Social and emotional well-being of workers

Supporting the social and emotional needs of staff entails responding to the emotional needs of workers when they feel overwhelmed, stressed or confused about their work (Mor Barak *et al*, 2009), as well as showing listening and empathy skills. In a study of hospice interdisciplinary team members in the US, DeLoach & Monroe (2004) report qualitative responses from open-ended survey questions on the aspects of supervision that staff found most supportive. Social and emotional support figured highly. For social workers, being supportive came in the form of feeling valued as a unique member of a specific discipline, being supported in clinical decision-making, and receiving supportive comments from supervisors that 'back you up'.

The provision of good quality, effective supervision is not just linked to the promotion of beneficial worker outcomes within the literature. The evidence also suggests that it may also help to mitigate against workers experiencing more negative detrimental outcomes such as stress, burnout or their intention to leave their employment. See Carpenter *et al* (2012) for a detailed summary of the literature also relating to the children and families context.

Five of the 14 studies looked at the association between supervision and intention to leave (Brannon *et al*, 2007; Fleming & Taylor, 2007; Kavanagh *et al*, 2003; Kim & Lee, 2009; Simons & Jankowski, 2007); all of which were conducted in interprofessional contexts. In a US study of direct care workers, Brannon *et al* (2007) reported that as respondents' assessment of quality of supervision increased, their intention to leave was reduced. Also the risk of being in the group with the highest intention to leave was reduced by 30% for each one point increase on the supervision measure, even when other factors were controlled for. Similar findings were reported by Simons and Jankowski (2007) in a US study of social workers based within nursing homes as part of a multidisciplinary care team. Workers who had increased supervisor and co-worker support showed decreased levels of quitting intent via increased job satisfaction and organisational commitment. Key study box 1 summarises findings from the only UK-based study included in the review.

Key study box 1: Fleming & Taylor (2007)

In the only UK based study to be included in the review, Fleming and Taylor (2007) adopt a mixed methods approach to explore the retention of home care workers (HCWs) in Northern Ireland from their own perspective. Based within an integrated health and social care service, 45 HCWs completed a written questionnaire, and focus groups with 12 HCWs were then used to look at emerging themes. The study was specifically aimed at social care workers who did not possess a social work qualification.

They reported that on the whole, HCWs were positive about supervision, with 80% stating that they felt they received sufficient support from their supervisor. However a significant minority did identify the need for more support. This included better communication, more responsive out-of-hours contact and emergency systems and additional support available at times of crisis, e.g. following the death of a client. Emergencies were a particular crunch point, with about a third of staff saying that they sometimes or never felt supported. A lack of management support was one of the main reasons given by HCWs for feeling dissatisfied and considering leaving, along with irregular and antisocial hours and workload pressures.

The authors concluded by highlighting the highly complex nature of the HCW's role, both in relation to clients' health needs and an increasingly regulated context in terms of quality and risk. This complexity adds to the demanding nature of the job and highlights the importance of good quality supervision and support. They added that the demands of the job role do not appear to be recognised in either the training or working conditions of staff, yet the factors identified in the paper give clear scope for service managers to improve the retention of HCWs, who are essential in providing a crucial healthcare service.

The degree to which supervisory support is associated with detrimental worker outcomes is subject to debate (Carpenter *et al*, 2012). Two of the 14 studies reviewed considered the effects of supervision on the detrimental worker outcomes of stress, burnout, secondary traumatisation and intention to leave (Ben-Porat & Itzhaky; Kim & Lee, 2009). Kim and Lee (2009) used statistical modelling to investigate the effects of different types of supervisory communication on burnout and intention to leave among 211 social workers in health or mental health settings in the US. They found that 'positive relationship communication', which they defined as informal and supportive interaction between supervisors and social workers, appeared to reduce worker stress and indirectly reduced burnout and intention to leave.

However, Ben-Porat and Itzhaky (2011) found that workers' satisfaction with supervision did not correlate significantly with either secondary traumatisation or burnout. This latter finding contradicts the theoretical literature, which argues that supervision is a substantial support system for workers in stressful situations, and highlights the need to further examine how supervision may help workers to combat the stressful job role.

Supervision and outcomes for organisations

Growing interest in the impact of supervision for organisations reflects both current pressures on agencies to ensure that services are cost effective, as well as a desire by researchers to better understand social work organisations and the staff who work there (Yoo, 2002). Three of the 14 studies explored the impact of supervision on organisational outcomes (Ben-Porat & Itzhaky, 2011; Bowers & Jacobson, 2002; Kavanagh *et al*, 2003). These studies present findings relating to the impact of supervision on either a workers' job performance or their perceived role competence.

Bowers & Jacobson (2002) conducted a small-scale study in the US exploring the impact of supervision on a worker's job performance. They reported that of all the conditions mentioned by practitioners as necessary for excellent practice, greatest emphasis was placed on having a supervisor who was supportive and facilitating, and that good supervisors were seen as 'collaborators' rather then 'overseers'.

A further study by Kavanagh *et al* (2003) (see Key study box 2) of social workers, psychologists and occupational therapists working in integrated mental health services found that their satisfaction with supervision and positive attitudes to supervisors were strongly associated with perceived impact on the effectiveness of their practice. A minority of these practitioners were supervised by someone from another discipline in the team, which enabled the researchers to compare perceptions of same-discipline and cross-discipline supervision.

According to the supervisees, the primary focus of supervision was discipline specific (46%) followed by generic practice (25%). The researchers reported that more time spent on discipline-specific skills was correlated with greater perceived impact on effectiveness, but time spent on generic skills was not. Frequency of contact was also important for supervisees' perceived impact on practice— the more frequent the contact with a supervisor of the same discipline the greater the perceived impact on clinical effectiveness, but there was no statistically significant relationship if supervisors were from a different discipline. As Kavanagh *et al* (2003) go on to suggest, this may indicate that certain features of supervision, such as direct instruction and skills acquisition, are particularly important, as was a perceived need to retain a discipline-specific focus in supervision sessions.

Key study box 2: Kavanagh *et al* (2003)

This study examined whether supervision characteristics impacted on the practice and morale of workers. A new survey entitled the 'Supervision Attitude Scale' (SAS) was developed for this study, and administered over the telephone to 272 staff from integrated public mental health services across Queensland, Australia, including social workers, psychologists and occupational therapists.

They reported that supervision was widely received by staff and largely rated positively, although some workers did raise concerns about the infrequency of sessions, and the availability and level of their supervisor's experience. Supervision was typically delivered in person using a one-to-one model (with teleconferencing used in some rural areas) and staff received a monthly (median) average of two hours. A minority of the participants were supervised by a supervisor from another discipline in the team which also enabled the researchers to compare perceptions of same-discipline and cross-discipline supervision.

According to the supervisees, the primary focus of supervision was discipline specific (46%) followed by generic practice (25%). The researchers reported that greater time spent on discipline-specific skills was correlated with greater perceived impact on effectiveness, but time spent on generic skills was not. Frequency of contact was also important for supervisee's perceived impact on practice—the more frequent the contact with a supervisor of the same discipline the greater the perceived impact on clinical effectiveness, but there was no statistically significant relationship if supervisors were from a different discipline.

The authors concluded '*positivity of the supervision relationship emerged as a key feature of effective supervision, both in terms of its impact on practice and on job satisfaction*' and thus this study supports the role of supervision in improving both retention and practice. The authors also go on to suggest that certain features of supervision (such as direct instruction and skills acquisition) are particularly important, as was a perceived need to retain a discipline-specific focus in supervision sessions.

Ben-Porat & Itzhaky (2011) also considered the potential impact of supervision on workers' perceived role competence. They reported that satisfaction with supervision correlated positively and significantly with two components of role competence: general competence and knowledge and problem-solving.

Although the supervision of social workers has increasingly focused on performance management, aiming to ensure that organisational procedures are followed and that staff are practising within agency expectations, there is very little research evidence that supervision actually affects a worker's job performance or role competence. While there may be an association between supervision and workers' perceptions of job performance or role competence in general, no studies actually evaluated the impact of supervision on either of these aspects.

Nor did these studies provide sufficient details on the supervisory process itself to allow for any conclusions to be drawn on how supervision positively affects job performance or role competence. It may be that the task assistance function of

supervision has a direct impact on workers' performance, but equally increased worker perceptions of their job performance or sense of role competence may be an indirect effect of supervision promoting a worker's self-efficacy—this is the difficulty of relying on correlational evidence.

Further, these studies only focused on organisational outcomes relating to the administrative or case management function of supervision. Yet there are undoubtedly additional organisational factors where supervision may also have an impact, such as workers' perceived organisational support or actual turnover and retention. This means that in order to understand the wider functions of supervision, we are forced to rely on evidence from studies relating to a children and families setting instead (e.g. Gonzalez *et al*, 2009; Landsman, 2008; Maertz *et al*, 2007).

Supervision and outcomes for service users and carers

There is a paucity of evidence on the impact of supervision on outcomes for service users and carers. Not one of the 14 studies discussed here investigated this. In part this reflects the difficulties of unravelling the distinct impact of supervision on service user outcomes, but it also reflects a preoccupation with outcomes for workers and organisations. This lack of evidence is not specific to the adult social work context, with only two studies in our wider systematic review making mention of the connection between supervision and outcomes for children and families (Collins-Camargo & Millar, 2010; Yoo, 2002).

This means that it is not possible to assess the impact of supervision on outcomes that matter to service users themselves, which may differ from policy and practice imperatives. It also means that any changes to the supervisory process are not informed by the perspectives of users and carers, and miss this crucial aspect to understanding how supervision affects practice. While not focused specifically on outcomes, Lambley & Marrable in chapter 5 of this volume report findings from service users themselves on supervision. They found that peoples' knowledge and understanding of supervision varied but that all considered it part of their overall service experience and hence they should have some influence over its development and delivery.

Conclusions, limitations and implications

→ Supervision appears to be typically delivered via an 'instrumental', one-to-one model, however all studies provided very few specific details about the supervisory process.

→ There is a distinct lack of intervention studies or those which consider models of group supervision within the adult social care literature, and all studies overlooked the concept of cost-effectiveness.

→ While 10 of the 14 studies were actually completed in inter-professional contexts, only two (Bogo *et al*, 2011a; 2011b) explore in any detail how supervision operates within an integrated setting. Where interprofessional supervision did occur staff had mixed reactions. Some workers missed the connection to their own professional discipline, but most felt that factors such as a safe and trusting supervisory relationship, along with a supervisor's clinical expertise and ability to provide relevant practice knowledge, were more important than professional affiliation.

→ Workers on multidisciplinary teams also value their colleagues as a source of feedback and support, but not at the expense of meeting with workers from their own profession.

→ Good supervision is associated with workers' job satisfaction (particularly where it is offered regularly, includes task-orientated advice and supports workers to access resources for clients), organisational commitment and their overall social and emotional well-being. However the complexities of workers' job roles and differing employment contexts must also be taken into account.

→ Supervisory support is also associated with reduced intention to leave, but mixed findings were found in relation to the impact on workers' stress, burnout and secondary traumatisation.

→ Supportive and facilitative supervisors are seen as necessary for excellent practice, and satisfaction with supervision is significantly associated with some aspects of role competence and workers' perceived impact on practice.

→ No studies explored the effects of supervision on service user or carer outcomes, and a lack of attention to these outcomes is also apparent within the wider social work literature. This may reflect a pre-occupation with worker and organisational outcomes, as well as difficulties in unravelling the specific impact of supervision on service users.

→ Similar to the children and families context, the empirical basis for supervision in adult social work and social care in the UK is weak. Most of the evidence is correlational and stems from services in the US.

Research clearly offers some valuable insights into the relationship between supervision and positive outcomes for workers and organisations. Yet as Carpenter *et al* (2013) state, *'given the insubstantial theoretical foundations, the lack of clearly defined models and the paucity of good evidence, "supervision" has a long way to go to prove itself as an evidence-based practice.'* This is especially true when considering supervision from a UK perspective: so few studies are UK-based it is difficult to draw out conclusions for a topic that is strongly connected to sector and organisational cultures.

Lack of evidence also makes it difficult to comment on the impact of interprofessional supervision on outcomes. Although some studies did attempt to explore the interprofessional supervisory relationship in more detail, findings were mixed. Gaining a more sophisticated understanding of the specific tensions involved in interprofessional supervision, such as upholding core values or imparting profession-specific knowledge, will help us to understand if there are key supervisory ingredients which supervisors need to deliver that would maximise the effectiveness of these arrangements.

References

Allen RI, Lambert EG, Pasupuleti S, Tolar TC & Ventura LA (2004) The impact of job characteristics on social and human service workers. *Social Work and Society* **2** (2) 173–188.

Ben-Porat A & Itzhaky H (2011) The contribution of training and supervision to perceived role competence, secondary traumatization, and burnout among domestic violence therapists. *The Clinical Supervisor* **30** (1) 95–108.

Bogo M, Paterson J, Tufford L & King R (2011a) Supporting front-line practitioners' professional development and job satisfaction in mental health and addiction. *Journal of Interprofessional Care* **25** (3) 209–214.

Bogo M, Paterson J, Tufford L & King R (2011b) Interprofessional clinical supervision in mental health and addiction: toward identifying common elements. *The Clinical Supervisor* **30** (1) 124–140.

Bowers BJ & Jacobson N (2002) Best practice in long-term care case management: how excellent case managers do their jobs. *Journal of Social Work in Long-Term Care* **1** (3) 55–72.

Bradley G & Höjer S (2009) Supervision reviewed: reflections on two different social work models in England and Sweden. *European Journal of Social Work* **12** 71–85.

Brannon D, Barry T, Kemper P, Schreiner A & Vasey J (2007) Job perceptions and intent to leave among direct care workers: evidence from the Better Jobs Better Care demonstration. *The Gerontologist* **47** (6) 820–829.

British Association of Social Workers and The College of Social Work (2011) *Research on Supervision in Social Work, with Special Reference to Social Workers Working in Multidisciplinary Teams* [online]. Available at: http://cdn.basw.co.uk/upload/basw_13955-1. pdf (accessed November 2015).

Cameron A, Lart R, Bostock L & Coomber C (2012) *Research Briefing 41: Factors that promote and hinder joint working in health and social care*. London: Social Care Institute for Excellence (SCIE).

Carpenter J, Webb CM & Bostock L (2013) The surprisingly weak evidence base for supervision: findings from a systematic review of research in child welfare practice (2000–2012). *Children and Youth Services Review* **35** 1843–1853.

Carpenter J, Webb CM, Bostock L & Coomber C (2012) *Research Briefing 43: Effective supervision in social work and social care*. London: SCIE.

Cole D, Panchanadeswaran S & Daining C (2004) Predictors of job satisfaction of licensed social workers: perceived efficacy as a mediator of the relationship between workload and job satisfaction. *Journal of Social Service Research* **31** (1) 1–12.

Collins-Camargo C & Millar K (2010) The potential for a more clinical approach to child welfare supervision to promote practice and case outcomes: a qualitative study in four states. *The Clinical Supervisor* **29** (2) 164–187.

DeLoach R & Monroe J (2004) Job satisfaction among hospice workers: what managers need to know. *Health Care Manager* **23** (3) 209–219.

Department for Children, Schools & Families (DCSF) (2009) *Facing Up to the Task: The interim report of the Social Work Task Force*. London: DCSF.

Egan M & Kadushin G (2004) Job satisfaction of home health social workers in the environment of cost containment. *Health and Social Work* **29** (4) 287–296.

Fleming G & Taylor BJ (2007) Battle on the home care front: perceptions of home care workers of factors influencing staff retention in Northern Ireland. *Health and Social Care in the Community* **15** (1) 67–76.

Gonzalez RP, Faller KC, Ortega RM & Tropman J (2009) Exit interviews of child welfare workers. *Journal of Public Child Welfare* **3** (1) 40-63.

Kavanagh DJ, Spence SH, Strong J, Wilson J, Sturk H & Crow N (2003) Supervision practices in allied mental health: relationships of supervision characteristics to perceived impact and job satisfaction. *Mental Health Services Research* **5** (4) 187–195.

Kim H & Lee SY (2009) Supervisory communication, burnout, and turnover intention among social workers in health care settings. *Social Work in Health Care* **48** (4) 364–385.

Landsman MJ (2008) Pathways to organizational commitment. *Administration in Social Work* **32** (2) 105–132.

Lee CD & del Carmen Montiel E (2011) The correlation of mentoring and job satisfaction: a pilot study of mental health professionals. *Community Mental Health Journal* **47** (4) 482–487.

Maertz CP Jr, Griffeth RW, Campbell NS & Allen DG (2007) The effects of perceived organizational support and perceived supervisor support on employee turnover. *Journal of Organizational Behavior* **28** (8) 1059–1075.

Manthorpe J, Moriarty J, Hussein S, Stevens M & Sharpe E (2013) Content and purpose of supervision in social work practice in England: views of newly qualified social workers, managers and directors. *British Journal of Social Work* **45** (1) 52-68.

Mor Barak ME, Travis DA, Pyun H & Xie B (2009) The impact of supervision on worker outcomes: a meta-analysis. *Social Service Review* **83** (1) 3–32.

Simons KV & Jankowski TB (2007) Factors influencing nursing home social workers' intentions to quit employment. *Administration in Social Work* **32** (1) 5–21.

Webb, CM & Carpenter J (2012) What Can Be Done to Promote the Retention of Social Workers? A Systematic Review of Interventions. *British Journal of Social Work* **42** 1235-55.

Yoo J (2002) The relationship between organizational variables and client outcomes: a case study in child welfare. *Administration in Social Work* **26** (2) 39–61.

Appendix: Summary of key research studies

	Authors	Study design	Participants	Method and description of supervision	Key reported outcomes	
					Worker	**Organisation**
1	Allen *et al* (2004)	Quantitative (cross-sectional)	Social workers and human services workers in the US (N = 255; actual respondents).	Survey measure used. Supervision not defined but was measured using 10 items from a variety of sources.	Job satisfaction, organisational commitment	N/A
2	Ben-Porat & Itzhaky (2011)	Quantitative (cross-sectional)	Social workers in Israel (N = 143; 70% response rate).	Survey measure used. Supervision not defined but was measured using the 'Multifactor Leadership Questionnaire'.	Burnout, secondary traumatisation	Role competence
3	Bogo *et al* (2011a)	Qualitative	Social workers, nurses and occupational therapists in Canada (N = 76).	13 focus groups completed and transcribed. Supervision described as monthly clinical supervision within an integrated setting. Supervision provided by either programme manager (from any profession) or designated advanced clinician/nurse.	Job satisfaction	N/A
4	Bogo *et al* (2011b)	Qualitative	Social workers, nurses and occupational therapists in Canada (N = 77).	14 focus groups completed and transcribed. Supervision described as clinical supervision delivered individually or via a group within an integrated setting. 38% reported supervision provided by supervisor from a different profession.	Job satisfaction	N/A
5	Bowers & Jacobson (2002)	Qualitative	Social workers in the US (N = 16).	Unstructured interviews with six 'excellent' case managers compared with ten 'very good' and 'good enough' case managers. Supervision not defined. Set in an interprofessional context.	N/A	Job performance

	Authors	Study design	Participants	Method and description of supervision	Key reported outcomes	
					Worker	Organisation
6	Brannon *et al* (2007)	Quantitative (cross-sectional)	Direct care workers in the US (N = 3,039; actual respondents with complete data).	Survey measure used (86-item BJBC Direct Care Worker Survey). Supervision not defined but responses focused on quality of supervision received (support and structure). Set in an interprofessional context.	Intention to leave	N/A
7	Cole *et al* (2004)	Quantitative (cross-sectional)	Social workers in the US (N = 232; actual respondents).	Survey measure used. Supervision not defined but responses focused on perceived quality of supervision received.	Job satisfaction	N/A
8	DeLoach & Monroe (2004)	Mixed Methods (quantitative & qualitative data)	Social workers, nurses, spiritual care providers & home health aides in the US (N = 72; actual respondents).	Questionnaire survey consisting of open-ended questions. Supervision not defined. Set in an interprofessional context.	Job satisfaction	N/A
9	Egan & Kadushin (2004)	Quantitative (cross-sectional)	Home health social workers in the US (N = 228; useable responses).	Survey measure used. Supervision not defined. Set in an interprofessional context.	Job satisfaction	N/A
10	Fleming & Taylor (2007)	Mixed Methods (quantitative & qualitative data)	Home care workers in the UK (N = 45 actual survey respondents & N = 12 focus group participants).	Survey measure examining training and induction, supervision and support and workers' feelings regarding the work. Focus groups used to explore emerging themes. Supervision not defined. Set in an interprofessional context.	Intention to leave	N/A
11	Kavanagh *et al* (2003)	Quantitative (cross-sectional)	Social workers, psychologists, occupational therapists and speech therapists in Australia (N = 272).	Telephone survey administered. Survey measure included newly designed Supervision Attitude Scale (SAS). Questions explored the frequency, focus and delivery of supervision. Set in an interprofessional context.	Job satisfaction, intention to leave	Job performance
12	Kim & Lee (2009)	Quantitative (cross-sectional).	Social workers in health or mental health settings in the US (N = 211).	Survey measure examining supervisory communication, role stress, burnout and turnover intention. Supervision not defined but supervisory communication consisted of job-relevant communication, upward communication, and positive relationship communication. Set in an interprofessional context.	Burnout, stress, intention to leave	N/A
13	Lee & del Carmen Montiel (2011)	Quantitative (cross-sectional)	Practitioners and supervisors in a mental health setting in the US (N = 56)	Online survey measure exploring job satisfaction and mentoring relationships. Focus on 'mentoring' rather than supervision. Different functions of the mentoring task acknowledged: sponsoring, assigning challenging tasks, and demonstrating trust.	Job satisfaction	N/A
14	Simons & Jankowski (2007)	Quantitative (cross-sectional)	Social workers in a health care (nursing home) setting in the US (N = 299; actual respondents)	Survey measure sent to directors of social work or social services at nursing facilities. Survey comprised of various measures with four items relating to supervisor support. Set in an interprofessional context.	Job satisfaction, intention to leave, organisational commitment	N/A

Chapter 3

Interprofessional clinical supervision of staff in mental health and addiction: Do common elements exist across professions?

Professor Marion Bogo and **Jane Paterson**

Introduction

Social work and related mental health professions have traditionally provided clinical supervision to members of their own profession. While there is some variation in definitions between professions, a generally accepted view is that clinical supervision is a process to address agency accountability for effective service and positive outcomes for clients, through a senior staff member providing support, professional development and guidance for the work of junior colleagues (Butterworth & Faugier, 2013; Gaitskill & Morley, 2008; Hall & Cox, 2009; Kadushin & Harkness, 2014; Milne, 2007). Traditionally, supervision is provided by senior members of the same profession as that of the front-line practitioner. New organisational arrangements in mental health and addiction services have led to supervision offered by those from a profession different from the supervisee, commonly referred to as interprofessional supervision (IPS).

A growing body of research across a variety of professions has identified the benefits of supervision, particularly for staff members. Studies show that clinical supervision can increase practitioners' sense of professional competence and job satisfaction (Knudsen et al, 2008; Schroffel, 1999; Strong et al, 2003), increase effective use of empirically supported treatments (Fixsen et al, 2009; Hoge et al, 2011), increase commitment to the organisation (MorBarak et al, 2009) and mediate organisational and professional stress as a result of restructuring and working in multiprofessional environments (Lloyd et al, 2002; Reid et al, 1999; Taylor & Bentley, 2005).

Publically funded health systems such as those in Canada and the UK must provide cost-effective service, often in the face of fewer resources to meet increasing and complex needs of populations. In addition, in semi-private systems (such as in the US) more efficient approaches are constantly sought

and a frequent response is to develop new organisational arrangements (Bazzoli et al, 2004; Burns et al, 2012). One outcome of such reorganisation initiatives in Canada was the elimination of profession-specific central departments replaced with programme management structures (Globerman et al, 2002). In these arrangements clinical supervision may be totally eliminated or provided by professionals from disciplines that are not the same as the practitioner. There is growing research literature that examines the nature and impact of this form of IPS. Davys and Beddoe provide a summary and analysis of studies in chapter 4.

The study reviewed in this chapter was conducted at the Centre for Addiction and Mental Health (CAMH), an organisation that had recently become the amalgamation of four organisations, thus becoming Canada's largest mental health and addiction teaching hospital, and one of the world's leading research centres (Bogo et al, 2011a; 2011b). Clients are people living and working in the community with serious, persistent mental illness and substance use. In addition, there is a large forensic population of individuals with mental illness who have been charged with a criminal offence. Organisation restructuring included the elimination of central professional departments that provided supervision to their staff and adoption of a programme management approach with supervision from managers or specially appointed supervisors (often from a profession different from that of the practitioner).

This chapter summarises the study's key findings with respect to the common elements of quality clinical supervision identified by practitioners across professions, and thus provides guidelines for those providing IPS. The study highlighted that supervision occurs in a context – that of the team and the organisation – and is powerfully affected by multilevel dimensions.

Method

Given the paucity of empirically-based knowledge about IPS, in the interests of developing a more in-depth understanding of the dynamics and impact of this approach, an exploratory study was deemed appropriate to uncover underlying and often hidden perspectives that could contribute to improving current supervisory practice. A form of qualitative data analysis that draws on some elements of grounded theory methods was used (Charmaz, 2006; Tweed & Charmaz, 2011).

Recruitment

Following approval by CAMH's research ethics board, staff were recruited via email, posters and presentations by the research assistants at team and profession-specific meetings. At that time the centre employed approximately 611 front-line staff from nursing, social work, occupational therapy, recreation therapy, child and youth work and stress management work. Seventy-six practitioners attended 14 focus groups. Participants included 22 nurses, 29 social workers, five occupational therapists, 10 recreation therapists, nine child and youth workers and one stress management therapist. Since psychiatrists do not receive supervision they were not included in this study. Of the participants, 62 worked in mental health programmes and 14 in addictions programmes.

Data collection

Two research assistants who were not known to the participants used a semi-structured interview to guide discussion in 14 focus groups of approximately two hours in duration. Discussions addressed practitioners' experiences, with, and perceptions of, clinical supervision, opportunities, facilitators and obstacles. The focus group meetings were all digitally recorded, then transcribed and anonymised. A software program was used for data management (QSRNUD_IST Vivo, 1999).

Data analysis

After conducting three initial focus groups, these transcripts were read independently by three members of the research team who used brief descriptors to identify codes. Constant comparative coding was then used in regular meetings to discuss the independent coding and to arrive at a draft coding framework. After four additional focus groups were held this coding framework was used for analysis. As coding progressed modifications were made resulting in refinement of codes and organisation into categories. During data analysis, two emerging themes led to refinements in the design. Firstly, participants spoke about IPS as only one aspect of enhancing job performance, competence and satisfaction. Important additional factors were the nature of the team and the organisation. Accordingly, subsequent interviews included questions about these dimensions. Secondly, some participating nurses expressed opinions about receiving supervision that differed markedly from other nurses and members of other professions. Although we actively tried to recruit more nurse participants to elaborate on this emerging category, the final sample remained small. As preliminary findings were emerging the research team met twice with current supervisors who constituted a project advisory committee to present and discuss emerging themes.

Results

Common elements

Three interrelated components of IPS emerged that were associated with quality supervision; structure, process and content (Bogo et al, 2011a). With respect to structure, participants who had previously regularly scheduled same-profession supervision viewed such arrangements as ideal. In such sessions there is time to engage in in-depth analysis and reflection about case dynamics, clinical decisions, plus positive and negative aspects of one's own practice. Of value were supervisors who are generally present and involved in the daily practice. Such supervisors were seen as having firsthand knowledge of the practitioner's work and hence their feedback was seen as credible, both about client situations and the practitioner's competence. Another crucial dimension is the availability of the supervisor; participants, especially those working in inpatient settings, wanted easy access to supervisors when challenging situations occurred.

With respect to content, it is important to note that practitioners in this study were working with challenging populations in an organisation committed to providing evidence-based programmes that embraced the most effective approaches. As new models were developed, professional staff expressed their high levels of commitment to learning to effectively provide interventions that would result in improved patient outcomes. Hence, they respected supervisors who were perceived as knowledgeable and expert in emerging, as well as current, effective treatments. As others have found (MorBarak et al, 2009) content expertise was seen as a crucial dimension for supervisors.

In complex work environments with heavy caseloads, rapid intake and discharge case discussions, the focus is often on practical and administrative decisions. Participants commented that there is little time for reflection to identify gaps and issues in one's own practice, or to consider process dynamics and counter-transference. Practitioners were interested in their own professional identity and development, and viewed supervision as an ideal space to deconstruct their work and examine their subjective reactions. Some nurse participants noted that IPS now provided this focus in contrast to their previous experiences with same-profession supervision, which had tended to be more administratively oriented. The common valued supervisory element that emerged can be labelled as practitioner-centered, where participants are involved in constructing the topics to be covered and where they perceived the sessions to be relevant to their practice.

With respect to process, participants noted that sensitive issues arise, frequently stimulated by interactions with clients, and these issues provoke strong personal feelings and reactions. For example, in one group interview, nurses and social workers identified their desire to discuss clinical situations where they were critical of their own behaviour. They wanted to examine their own internal dynamics, reactions, culture or gender biases. A trusting relationship with the clinical supervisor was paramount for open, honest discussions of topics where they felt vulnerable. They hoped to gain some perspective about their sense of self-competence. In this respect, it was noted that safety and trust were more significant than whether supervisor and supervisee shared the same professional background.

Trusting relationships were characterised as providing both validation and critical comments. Since many client situations are not amenable to 'straightforward' interventions, front-line staff reported feelings of uncertainty and being overwhelmed. They valued supervisors who appreciated staff's efforts and commitments, but who could at the same time point out attitudes and behaviours that might be more effective in handling practice challenges.

Trusting relationships are also seen as reciprocal; feedback about performance is not only unidirectional. Engaged supervisors ask practitioners whether their supervision is useful and to provide information about what could be changed. This type of collaboration models a parallel process that practitioners can experience and then use with clients.

Exceptions

These perceptions about the structure, content and process of clinical supervision appeared to generally cross professions. They could be considered as universal elements of a supervision model. Some nurses, however, held different views from their nursing colleagues and those from other professions. These nurse participants were generally negative about supervision, based on examples within their own profession where supervision was experienced as punitive, hierarchical and invoked when a nurse was chastised for some activity needing correction. These negative perceptions led participants to be fearful and apprehensive of any supervision arrangements. Others did not perceive supervision as necessary for professionals who are self-regulated. They referred to their provincial regulatory body as recognising nurses as autonomous and self-reliant; they expected that each nurse had the responsibility to seek out consultation with appropriate individuals if they felt that the task they were doing was beyond their scope or level of competence.

An additional exception that arose from the discussions was that practitioners needed a somewhat different experience based on their stage of professional development. For example, new graduates needed orientation and connection to their own professions so that they could clearly understand unique features of their role. Additionally, they needed more educational input and support, especially if they were new to the organisation or to the treatment approach. Same-profession supervisors could provide mentoring, socialising and career guidance for the novice practitioner.

Experienced practitioners who were new members of the organisation expressed the need for information specific to effective functioning in their teams as they adapted their knowledge and skills to the new environment. Of interest was that nurses, social workers and occupational therapists, who were both experienced practitioners and longstanding members of the organisation, still believed that clinical supervision could add value to their practice. They observed that one could become complacent about practice. In supervision, long-held views and practices can be challenged and stimulate new learning. Moreover, one standard of the regulatory provincial body for nurses in this study states that nurses should not perform a task with which they are not comfortable. As new knowledge emerges and practice expectations change, organisations may offer workshops to assist staff in their practice. Implementation science however,

has shown that integrating new approaches into practice requires continuous clinical supervision focused on reinforcing new interventions (Fixsen et al, 2009).

Comparison of same-profession supervision and IPS

Practitioners in professions with well-established traditions of clinical supervision, such as social work, valued past arrangements as enhancing their professional learning and practice. The centre had recently provided clinical supervision for nurses offered by advanced practice nurses and these sessions were also received positively. New IPS was received variably, largely dependent on whether the previously noted common elements were present. Where supervisors were seen as not having the clinical and content expertise needed to assist the practitioner, it was felt the meetings were not as helpful. If the supervision was unfocused, unstructured and not perceived as clinically relevant, then it was not seen as helpful.

It was clear that practitioners wanted clinical supervision that was practitioner and client-centered and negatively viewed supervision that was more focused on administrative topics such as time management. For some participants the new clinical supervision arrangements represented a fresh and stimulating approach. Used to a more administrative focus, they welcomed the relational focus and collaborative style, including reflection on the staff member's experience. Mixed feelings were expressed about receiving supervision from those responsible for performance review. In the context of organisation downsizing, practitioners feared that if they were open about their practice challenges they would lose their jobs in the next round of cutbacks.

The common elements discussed earlier appeared to be the critical factor in whether IPS was experienced positively. Nevertheless, participants wanted the opportunity to connect with colleagues from their own profession. Such meetings provide a place and space to discuss new developments or changes in their profession and use their own professional language. Particularly for practitioners who are the lone representative of their profession on a team, being 'in the room' with others from the same profession provided a network for information sharing, future guidance and affirmation of one's profession-informed approach. Participants observed and valued those supervisors from another profession who tried to understand the unique frameworks and values of their supervisees. They noted however, that this requires considerable time and hence is not realistic in all circumstances.

The impact of context

Study participants underscored that supervision takes place in the context of teams and a complex organisation, the nature of which affects their work experience. These contextual dimensions also influence whether any type of supervision promotes quality practice and service to the population. Practitioners spontaneously discussed how they 'work and live' in their interprofessional teams in this organisation and the importance of informal support, joint review and planning activities. Learning resulted from this continuous interaction with stable, small, cohesive teams. That team members are in close daily proximity led to forming close connections which sustained professionalism and decreased isolation. Knowing that colleagues who could assist them in a crisis were nearby was seen as extremely important. Supervision could augment, but not replace, this important source of assistance and learning.

Participants freely expressed a range of opinions about what they referred to as 'the organisation'. Concerns about continuing downsizing and job security were shared, leading front-line staff to be reluctant to approach supervisors and managers too often with practice issues, fearing they would be seen as less competent and terminated in future job cuts. Of interest was the desire for a work environment that held staff accountable, but was not a blaming culture when mistakes occurred. As with clinical supervisors, programme managers were respected and valued if they were available, knowledgeable, helpful and effective team leaders. Managers with responsibility for performance review were only seen as credible if they had actually observed the practitioner's work over time. Finally, continuing education offered by the organisation was highly valued especially when it involved workshops on specialised treatment models or challenging daily issues. Mandatory training on topics not perceived as crucial for daily practice received less support from front-line staff.

Discussion

Similar to others' findings about clinical supervision, there are both positive and negative elements for staff (Milne *et al*, 2008; MorBarak *et al*, 2009). Common elements relate to the structure, content and process of supervision and these elements appear salient in both uniprofessional supervision and IPS. In summary, positive elements include availability, in regularly scheduled supervision and being onsite, as needed. Supervisors should have content expertise and skills relevant to the particular population. They must also be effective teachers; able to create and sustain a practitioner-centered approach. Such an approach provides a safe and open space to also consider personal/professional dynamics that impact practitioners' sense of self competence and also address professional development. The primacy of a reciprocal relationship with mutual feedback was seen as ideal. Negative elements involve focusing on administrative rather than clinical matters (not being perceived as clinically relevant) and a destructive, critical style emphasising practitioners' deficits. When positive elements were present in IPS, the new model did not negatively impact the study participants. Conversely, when these elements were present prior to the change, but no longer available in the new arrangements, IPS was viewed negatively.

Exceptions to these general principles emerged with novice practitioners needing connection to their own professions for orientation, socialisation and to develop role clarity in multiprofessional teams. Experienced practitioners also valued opportunities to discuss profession-specific issues but supervision was not necessarily the place for this. Regular profession-specific meetings could fill this gap. We concluded that the common elements in combination with profession-specific structures can meet practitioners' needs. Finally, some nurse practitioners viewed themselves as autonomous professionals, governed by their regulatory bodies and standards of practice, with the responsibility to identify gaps in practice and seek appropriate consultation.

Relevant to this discussion is whether IPS makes a difference with respect to client outcomes. In general, the research literature on the impact of supervision on client outcomes is scant. Recent reviews find considerable methodological weakness in the studies, limiting our ability to have confidence in the research. A recent review of the literature on supervision in publicly funded services in mental health and substance use services in the US found the majority of reports were conceptual or descriptive, largely exploratory, and few examined the association between supervision and client outcomes (Hoge *et al*, 2011). Outcome measures were self-reports by practitioners and agency directors. Indeed, a limitation of the study reported in this chapter is the use of self-report by practitioners. Similar methodological weakness was found in a recent review of the evidence base for clinical supervision in child welfare (Carpenter *et al*, 2013). The authors conclude that while associations between the provision of supervision and positive outcomes for workers exist, there are no reports of outcomes for service recipients.

There are however some examples of well-designed studies examining supervision with multidisciplinary staff (largely psychologists and social workers) using highly specific psychotherapy approaches. Some examples are reported by Lau *et al* (2004) using Trauma Focused Cognitive-Behavioural Therapy, by Henggeler *et al* (2002) using Multisystemic Family Therapy, and by Bambling *et al* (2006) using a supervision manual for experienced psychologists and social workers treating patients with major depression. Clearly there is a need to determine whether the elements identified for IPS by practitioners make a significant difference for client outcomes as well as for front-line workers.

References

Bambling M, King R, Raue P, Schweitzer R & Lambert W (2006) Clinical supervision: its influence on client-rated working alliance and client symptom reduction in the brief treatment of major depression. *Psychotherapy Research* **16** (3) 317–331.

Bazzoli GJ, Dynan L, Burns LR & Yap C (2004) Two decades of organisational change in health care: what have we learned? *Medical Care Research and Review* **61** (3) 247–331.

Bogo M, Paterson J, Tufford L & King R (2011a) Interprofessional clinical supervision in mental health and addiction: toward identifying common elements. *The Clinical Supervisor* **30** (1) 124–140.

Bogo M, Paterson J, Tufford L & King R (2011b) Supporting front-line practitioners' professional development and job satisfaction in mental health and addiction. *Journal of Interprofessional Care* **25** (3) 209–214.

Burns LR, Whaley DR, McCullough JS, Kralovec P & Muller R (2012) The changing configuration of hospital systems: centralisation federalisation or fragmentation. In: L Friedman, GT Savage & J Goes (Eds) *Annual Review of Health Care Management* (pp189–232). Bingley, UK: Emerald Group.

Butterworth T & Faugier J (2013) *Clinical Supervision and Mentorship in Nursing* (3rd edition). Cheltenham, UK: Nelson Thomas.

Carpenter J, Webb CM & Bostock L (2013) The surprisingly weak evidence base for supervision: findings from a systematic review of research in child welfare practice (2000 2012). *Children and Youth Services Review* **35** (11) 1843–1853.

Charmaz K (2006) *Constructing Grounded Theory: A practical guide through qualitative analysis*. Thousand Oaks, CA: SAGE.

Fixsen DL, Blase KA, Naoom SF & Wallace F (2009) Core implementation components. *Research on Social Work Practice* **19** (5) 531–540.

Gaitskill S & Morley M (2008) Supervision in occupational therapy: how are we doing? *British Journal of Occupational Therapy* **71** (3) 119–121.

Globerman J, White J & McDonald G (2002) Social work in restructuring hospitals: program management five years later. *Health & Social Work* **27** (4) 274–283.

Hall T & Cox D (2009) Clinical supervision: an appropriate term for physiotherapists? *Learning in Health and Social Care* **8** (4) 282–291.

Henggeler SW, Schoenwald SK, Liao JG, Letourneau EJ & Edwards DL (2002)Transporting efficacious treatments to field settings: the link between supervisory practices and therapist fidelity in MST programs. *Journal of Clinical Child and Adolescent Psychology* **31** (2) 155–167.

Hoge MA, Migdole S, Farkas MS, Ponce AN & Hunnicutt C (2011) Supervision in public Sector behavioral health: a review. *The Clinical Supervisor* **30** (2) 183–203.

Kadushin A & Harkness D (2014) *Supervision in social work* (5th edition). New York: Columbia University Press.

Knudsen HK, Ducharme LJ & Roman PM (2008) Clinical supervision emotional exhaustion and turnover intention: a study of substance abuse treatment counselors in the clinical trials network of the National Institute on Drug Abuse. *Journal of Substance Abuse Treatment* **35** (4) 387–395.

Lau M, Dubord GM & Parikh SV (2004) Design and fleasibility of a new cognitive behavioral course using a longitudinal interactive format. *The Canadian Journal of Psychiatry* **49** (10) 696–700.

Lloyd C, McKenna K & King R (2002) Social work stress and burnout: a review. *Journal of Mental Health* **11** (3) 255–265.

Milne D (2007) An empirical definition of clinical supervision. *British Journal of Clinical Psychology* **46** (4) 437–447.

Milne D, Aylott H, Fitzpatrick H & Ellis MV (2008) How does clinical supervision work? Using a 'best evidence synthesis' approach to construct a basic model of supervision. *The Clinical Supervisor* **27** (2) 170–190.

MorBarak ME, Travis DJ, Pyun H & Xie B (2009) The impact of supervision on worker outcomes: a meta-analysis. *Social Service Review* **83** (1) 3–32.

Reid Y, Johnson S, Morant N, Kuipers E, Smuckler G, Thornicroft G & Prosser D (1999) Explanations for stress and satisfaction in mental health professions: a qualitative study. *Social Psychiatry and Psychiatric Epidemiology* **34** 301–308 .

Schroffel A (1999) How does clinical supervision affect job satisfaction? *The Clinical Supervisor* **18** (2) 91–105.

Strong J, Kavanagh D, Wilson J, Spense SH, Worrall L & Crow N (2003) Supervision practice for allied health professionals within a large mental heath service: exploring the phenomenon. *The Clinical Supervisor* **22** (1) 191–210.

Taylor MF & Bentley KJ (2005) Professional dissonance: colliding values and job tasks in mental health practice. *Community Mental Health Journal* **41** (4) 469–481.

Tweed A & Charmaz K (2011) Grounded theory methods for mental health practitioners. In: D Harper & A Thompson (Eds) *Qualitative Research Methods in Mental Health and Psychotherapy: A guide for students and practitioners* (pp131–147). Chichester: Wiley Blackwell.

Chapter 4

Interprofessional supervision: Opportunities and challenges

Allyson Davys and Professor Liz Beddoe

In the supervision literature there is often a general assumption that both supervisor and supervisee will be trained professionals in the same discipline, holding common codes of ethics, values, norms and professional aims. That this is not universal is indicated by the emergence of cross-disciplinary supervision, now most frequently referred to as interprofessional supervision (IPS). The developing practice of IPS is possibly more common in the supervision of practitioners who work in private practice or who work in adult services such as mental health, addictions, palliative care and so on. These latter contexts often involve multidisciplinary ways of working together to deliver services. Here teams have evolved with a lesser focus on highly rigid professional roles and a shared appreciation of the value of different perspectives. IPS is a relatively new phenomenon and research to date suggests there are both opportunities and challenges to the practice. This chapter examines the rationale for seeking IPS, the perceived opportunities and challenges for the supervisor and supervisee and explores some recent research. Suggestions will be made about good practice, reinforcing the importance of clarity of purpose, clear boundaries and expectations and a focus on relationship.

Professional supervision is a cornerstone of practice for many professionals working within the health and social service sectors and has a tradition of being conducted between practitioners from the same profession (Bernard & Goodyear, 2009). In recent years, however, literature reporting partnerships between a supervisor and a supervisee from different professions has increased, suggesting a growth in the practice (Beddoe & Howard, 2012; Townend, 2005). A range of terms have been used to describe this form of supervision including 'cross-disciplinary' (Hair, 2013; Hutchings *et al*, 2014; O'Donoghue, 2004; Simmons *et al*, 2007), 'multidisciplinary' (Gillig & Barr, 1999) and 'multiprofessional' (Mullarkey *et al*, 2001). In line with others (Bogo *et al*, 2011; Townend, 2005) and also in keeping with previous research by the authors (Beddoe & Howard, 2012; Davys & Beddoe, 2008) we have chosen to use the term 'interprofessional supervision'.

Townend (2005) provides the following definition of IPS.

'Two or more [practitioners] *meeting from different professional groups to achieve a common goal of protecting the welfare of the client. This protection is achieved through a process that enables increased knowledge, increased skill, appropriate attitude and values to maintain clinical and professional competence.'* (p586)

It is useful to note in this definition that supervision is described as a process, where the goal is to protect the service user.

Research on interprofessional supervision

To date few studies of IPS have been undertaken. Those that have been conducted have largely focused on the incidence and experience of IPS within specific professions (Beddoe & Howard, 2012; Berger & Mizrahi, 2001; Hair, 2013; Howard *et al*, 2013; Hutchings *et al*, 2014) or within specific practice contexts (Bogo *et al*, 2011; Strong *et al*, 2004; Townend, 2005). An exception to this is Crocket *et al* (2009) whose criterion for participation in the study was that the participant was a supervisor who was providing IPS, and was not specific as to profession or context.

Table 4.1 summarises research which has explored IPS over the past 15 years and provides a broad overview of the research data collection methods, the populations sampled and the work contexts. General findings regarding the incidence and experience of IPS are also included.

Key factors

The body of research summarised in Table 4.1 illuminates the growth of IPS. We believe four key factors can be considered as influencing this development and the increased popularity of this form of supervision. These factors encompass structural, organisational and accountability dimensions along with elements of professional choice.

Firstly, reform within health and social care organisations, driven by the political agenda to reduce costs in health and social services and create greater efficiency in an increasingly competitive market environment has brought about major restructuring. Management and supervisory positions which hitherto represented, managed and supported separate profession based departments have been rationalised or eliminated (Berger & Mizrahi, 2001). In the resulting flattened and generic structures, managers no longer automatically share the profession of their team members and supervisors do not necessarily share the profession of their supervisees (Berger & Mizrahi, 2001; Bogo *et al*, 2011).

Berger and Mizrahi (2001), noting these changes, explored the models of supervision used by social workers working in hospital settings in the US. Three surveys were conducted between 1992 and 1996. Whilst Berger and Mizrahi found that the traditional same-profession supervision arrangement was

Table 4.1: Research on IPS – a summary

Study	Method	Practice context	Professions	IPS supervision	Adjunctive modes of supervision
Beddoe & Howard (2012)	Survey: 423 respondents engaged in IPS (supervisors and supervisees).	Range of practice contexts (New Zealand)	Psychology, social work	All engaged in IPS. Overall very satisfied with the IPSIPS received.	Also receiving same profession supervision: 63.6% of psychologists 52.2% of social workers.
Berger & Mizrahi (2001)	Survey: 1992 & 1994: 340 respondents 1996: 311 respondents.	Hospital based social work (US)	Social work	1992 - 12% of respondents IPS, 1994 - 16.1% of respondents IPS, 1996 - 19% of respondents IPS.	Only receiving IPS: 1992: 7.2%, 1994: 8.4%, 1996: 10%.
Bogo et al (2011)	Focus groups: 77 volunteer clinicians.	Mental health (Canada)	Nursing, social work, occupational therapy, recreation therapy, case worker/ child and youth worker, stress management therapy.	'…supportive, clinician-focused, content-oriented supervision offered by knowledgeable and skilled clinical experts was perceived as beneficial, regardless of the supervisor's profession' (p.135).	Participants 'expressed a need to discuss profession-specific issues and learn about new trends.' (p.133)
Crocket et al (2009)	Semi structured interviews: six supervisors.	Health and private practice (New Zealand)	Social work, counselling, psychology	All provide IPS. Benefits identified for: practitioners and their practice, the practitioner's organisation and the supervisors (p.30).	No relevant data available.
Globerman et al (2002)	Telephone survey: 12 sites in 1995. Expanded to 21 sites in 1999 due to amalgamation. Senior social worker.	Hospital (Canada)	Social work	Lack of professional support systems (that is, social work directors or supervisors (p.277) social workers…described feeling lost and isolated from their profession (p.280)).	Rarely engaged in same profession supervision.
Hair (2013)	Survey: 636 respondents, social worker supervisees.	Broad spectrum of settings (Canada)	Social work	36% have IPS.	Strong recommendation for same profession supervision.
Hutchings et al (2014)	Survey: 54 respondents, social work practitioners.	Social work (New Zealand)	Social work	25.9% received IPS as supervisee, 29.6% provided IPS as supervisor, 44.5% were both supervisee and supervisor. On average reported they were satisfied with the supervision they received.	84.2% of supervisees had same profession supervision.
Strong et al (2004)	Focus groups: 58 practitioners. Telephone interviews: 21 managers.	Mental health (Australia)	Occupational therapy, social work, psychology, speech therapy.	Concern that IPS devalues discipline, specific skills and potential for clash of frameworks resulting in ethical dilemmas. IPS valuable so long as specific ground rules observed (p.202).	Supervisees should have access to discipline-specific supervision.
Townend (2005)	Survey: 170 supervisees.	Cognitive behavioural therapists (UK)	Psychiatry, mental health nursing, social work, psychology, general practice, teacher/lecturer, occupational therapy, counselling.	40% received IPS, 59% report IPS never gets in the way of supervision, 26% report IPS rarely gets in the way of supervision.	Only one respondent reported receiving both IPS and same profession supervision.

significantly more common, the incidence of supervision being provided by a supervisor from another profession rose from 12% to 19% during that time frame. In Canada, Globerman et al (2002) surveying social workers employed in Canadian hospitals which had adopted a programme management approach, report that by 1999 it was rare for social workers to be involved 'with colleagues in peer consultation and supervision' (p277).

Secondly, and closely associated with the first factor, interprofessional working through multidisciplinary teams has been promoted as affecting best service user outcomes. Although much has been reported regarding the difficulties inherent in this (Hudson, 2002; 2007; McCallin, 2001; Townend, 2005) some professionals have begun to value the supervision opportunities this brings. Specifically, in the mental health sector Townend (2005) found that IPS relationships brought an increased understanding of different professional roles and divisions of responsibility. Practitioners considered these to be of benefit to work within the multidisciplinary setting. Again in the mental health context, where health programmes were delivered in a programme management model through a multidisciplinary team structure, Bogo et al, (2011) found that 'participants identified teams as a central support for practice' (p133). In this setting, team supervisors who were 'skilled at promoting cohesion, which in turn leads to engaged discussion and problem solving' (p133) were valued.

Thirdly, in increasingly regulated practice environments, governments and the public require assurance regarding the competence of health and social service practitioners. In some settings supervision has been introduced and employed as a means of ensuring safe practice in a risk averse climate (Beddoe, 2010). The pressure that this has put on the existing pools of supervisors has meant that some practitioners have had to go beyond their own profession to secure the required supervision (Beddoe & Howard, 2012).

Finally, in order to meet the demands of changing and complex practice contexts, a number of practitioners choose a supervisor because of that supervisor's particular skills and knowledge rather than because of his or her professional affiliation (Beddoe & Howard, 2012; Bogo et al, 2011; Hutchings et al, 2014; Townend, 2005). This is a choice often accompanied and influenced by a growing discernment on the part of the practitioner of the supervisor's supervision skills and the quality of supervision delivered. The respondents of the research conducted by Bogo et al (2011) who included nurses, social workers, occupational therapists, recreation therapists, child and youth workers and stress management therapists, 'almost universally' agreed that supervisors were valued because of their relational skills, their expertise as both supervisors and practitioners and their ability to facilitate learning. These qualities of the supervisor were seen as more important than the supervisor's professional affiliation.

When left to choose their supervisor, practitioners demonstrate that they are not necessarily bound by traditional same-profession supervision and will select a supervisor who they believe best meets their needs regardless of that person's profession. In a study of the IPS experiences of social workers in Aotearoa, New Zealand, Hutchings et al (2014) found that 91% of the supervisees they surveyed 'had influence over who provided their cross-disciplinary supervision' (p58). Choice has been identified in other studies as an important factor

in creating good supervision relationships (Bond & Holland, 2010; Davys, 2003) and as Scaife (2009) notes 'when choice is possible there is a view that experienced practitioners benefit more from the challenge and stimulation of a new approach rather than gravitation towards the familiar' (p19). By choosing IPS, practitioners would appear to be embracing the opportunity and challenge of difference. Indeed, in several studies participants have voiced their appreciation of the value of a different external perspective and critique when reflecting on and reviewing their practice (Howard et al, 2013; Hutchings et al, 2014; Townend, 2005). Rains (2007) introduces another perspective when reporting that some nursing practitioners viewed IPS as a means of addressing the legacy of historic 'hierarchical models of supervision' (p65). In a study of social workers and psychologists who participated in IPS, Howard et al (2013) record that the majority of supervisees (52.4%) considered the supervisor's knowledge and skills to have influenced their choice of supervisor. Almost 43% of the supervisees chose their supervisor because of the supervisor's understanding and knowledge of the work context and 22.9% because of a previous positive relationship with that person. The study also reports that one third accessed IPS because of a lack of available or appropriate supervisors in their own profession (Howard et al, 2013).

The opportunities and challenges

The benefits of IPS as reported in the research literature focus on three areas. The development of skills and knowledge (Beddoe & Howard, 2012; Townend, 2005), an awakening to the assumptions of practice and the development of critical thinking (Bogo et al, 2011; Hutchings et al, 2014) and a better understanding and appreciation of the different professional contributions, perspectives and roles in practice settings (Howard et al, 2013; Mullarkey et al, 2001).

Thus, IPS provides an opportunity for practitioners to explore their practice through the facilitation of another professional who, through his or her difference, can offer fresh and rich perspectives, introduce new and different knowledge and skill sets and can challenge the 'taken for granted' assumptions which creep into daily practice. An understanding can also be gained of the different roles and the potential contributions of other professionals which in turn lead to enhanced practice relationships and ultimately better service to consumers.

The challenges of IPS mirror the benefits. Where difference can be regarded as an advantage or an opportunity for growth, the flip side reveals possible limitations. The concerns reported in the literature about the practice of IPS can also be grouped into three themes. The first and possibly the most prevalent concern is the management of difference: knowledge, values, skills and professional contexts (Bogo et al, 2011; Howard et al, 2013; Townend, 2005). The second concern relates to the first and identifies the difficulty of managing different ethical and practice codes and reporting on profession-based competencies (Beddoe & Howard, 2012; Crocket et al, 2009; Hutchings et al, 2014). Finally, the literature registers concern that IPS will lead to a weakening of socialisation to a particular profession and thus a weakening of distinct professional identity (Berger & Mizrahi, 2001; Bernard & Goodyear, 2009; Hair, 2013).

Discussion and recommendations

Interestingly, despite the concerns noted above, studies on IPS report that the participants are by and large satisfied by the supervision they receive (Howard *et al*, 2013; Hutchings *et al*, 2014; Townend, 2005). One study notes that the qualities of the supervisor and the quality of the supervision provided were valued over and above professional affiliation.

'Supportive, clinician-focused, content-oriented supervision offered by knowledgeable and skilled clinical experts was perceived as beneficial, regardless of the supervisor's profession. Supervisors' expertise regarding the client population and effective interventions, as well as their ability to promote learning and a sense of competence for clinicians, emerged as highly valued.' (Bogo *et al*, 2011, p135)

That being said, IPS has been received differently by different professions and practitioners within those professions. In social work, where there is a long tradition of same-profession supervision, IPS has been reported by some researchers with alarm (Berger & Mizrahi, 2001) and regarded as an example of professional erosion (Hair, 2013). In contrast other studies, which have also included social workers, suggest a high incidence of social workers choosing to be supervised by a person from a different profession (Beddoe & Howard, 2012, Hutching *et al*, 2014).

Although opinion remains divided, the research literature offers useful comments and recommendations regarding the practice of IPS. These recommendations, when considered together, suggest the beginnings of a set of guidelines which we have assembled to assist those embarking on IPS.

Firstly some broad considerations as to who is best suited to engage in IPS. IPS is not recommended for everyone, and we support the general agreement in the literature that students, new graduates and practitioners who are new to an area or context of practice, are best supervised by a person from their own profession. We also agree that IPS is inappropriate where there is an identified performance issue. Whether IPS is sufficient on its own for other practitioners, or whether it should be in parallel with supervision from a supervisor within that practitioner's profession, is a matter for debate. In this regard what is important is that there is discussion as to where and how the practitioner accesses profession-specific advice and critique, and how different lines of accountability are managed.

Secondly, the contracting process, critical to all supervision relationships, brings additional considerations when it involves negotiating a contract across professions. The supervision contract needs to consider the totality of the practitioner's work, their varied professional and organisational accountabilities and to realistically and honestly identify any limitations of the interprofessional arrangement and how these can be addressed. The contracting process provides the forum for all these beginning conversations and will shape the eventual parameters and expectations of the supervision relationship.

The contracting conversation thus needs to ensure that the participants spend sufficient time exploring and understanding the differences that they bring to the relationship. These will include not only different professional codes, ethics and accountability structures, but also practice experience, knowledge and theoretical position. Also important is an exploration of each participant's approach to supervision and the key functions to be addressed in this particular interprofessional relationship. Models of supervision commonly describe three functions: the administrative/managerial, the educative and the supportive. The participants in interprofessional arrangements need to identify which functions will be attended to within supervision and how and where those not attended to will be addressed.

Underpinning these guidelines is a subtext which emphasises the process of IPS as much as the content: open and honest dialogue, exploration of difference, understanding of what each participant brings to the relationship and what each participant wants from the relationship. We highlight the importance of a robust process for establishing the supervision contract with commitment to regular review of the supervision activities, relationship and the agreed contract.

Table 4.2 identifies a set of questions to guide the conversation between the supervisor and supervisee when establishing the relationship and the supervision contract.

Table 4.2: Preparing for IPS	
1.	What is each participant's professional training and practice experience?
2.	What theoretical framework is used in practice by each party and what does this mean for supervision?
3.	How does each participant view the supervision process, what model of supervision will be used and what supervision functions will IPS address?
4.	How will the supervisee address any supervision functions not covered?
5.	What does the supervisee want from IPS?
6.	What are the supervisee's professional development and supervision goals?
7.	What expectations do the supervisee and supervisor have of each other?
8.	If there is disagreement, how will this be resolved?
9.	What actual or perceived differences of status are there between supervisor and supervisee? How will they be noticed and managed?
10.	What professional codes, values and ethics does each party bring to the relationship? What does this mean for supervision?
11.	Who has clinical responsibility for the supervisee's practice?
12.	To whom is the supervisee professionally accountable?
13.	To whom is the supervisee organisationally accountable?
14.	What relationship does this supervision arrangement have to 10, 11 and 12 above?
15.	Do the supervisee and supervisor agree that the supervisor has sufficient knowledge and expertise to provide supervision in this instance?
16.	If there is a question or issue which arises in supervision that requires profession-specific knowledge, who will be approached?
17.	What records will be kept and who will have access to them?
18.	When and how will the supervision process and contract be reviewed?
19.	What other differences might affect this relationship?

Summary

IPS, as the title of this chapter notes, brings both challenges and opportunities. It challenges some firmly held beliefs about the uniqueness of professional knowledge and expertise and brings into relief the range of accountability and responsibility held by individual practitioners. The opportunities can also be challenging as practitioners move from their known fields and present their work for reflection and critique to the outside eye. If, however, like Townend (2005), we view the goal of IPS to be for the welfare of the service user through increased professional competence, then the benefits of IPS are clear. This is well summed up in the comment of a social worker participant in Hair's (2013) study: *'by advocating to be profession specific we are overlooking the thing that makes our role strong: diversity of skills, of approach, of perspectives.'* (p1579).

References

Beddoe L (2010) Surveillance or reflection: professional supervision in 'the risk society'. *British Journal of Social Work* **40** (4) 1279–1296.

Beddoe L & Howard F (2012) Interprofessional supervision in social work and psychology: mandates and (inter)professional relationships. *The Clinical Supervisor* **31** (2) 178–202.

Berger C & Mizrahi T (2001) An evolving paradigm of supervision within a changing health care environment. *Social Work in Health Care* **32** (4) 1–18.

Bernard JM & Goodyear R (2009) *Fundamentals of Clinical Supervision* (4th edition). Upper Saddle River, NJ: Pearson.

Bogo M, Paterson J, Tufford L & King R (2011) Interprofessional clinical supervision in mental health and addiction: toward identifying common elements. *The Clinical Supervisor* **30** (1) 124–140.

Bond M & Holland M (2010) *Skills of Clinical Supervision for Nurses* (2nd edition). Maidenhead: Open University Press.

Crocket K, Cahill F, Flanagan P, Franklin J, McGill, R Stewart A, Whalan M & Mulcahy D (2009) Possibilities and limits of cross-disciplinary supervision. *New Zealand Journal of Counselling,* **29** (2) 25–43.

Davys A (2003) *Perceptions Through a Prism: Three accounts of good supervision*. Unpublished Master of Social Work thesis. Massey University, New Zealand.

Davys A & Beddoe L (2008) Interprofessional learning for supervision: 'taking the blinkers off'. *Learning in Health and Social Care* **8** (1) 58–69.

Gillig PM & Barr A (1999) A model for multidisciplinary peer review and supervision of behavioral health clinicians. *Community Mental Health Journal* **35** (4) 361–365.

Globerman J, White J & McDonald G (2002) Social work in restructuring hospitals: program management five years later. *Health and Social Work* **27** (4) 274–284.

Hair HJ (2013) The purpose and duration of supervision, and the training and discipline of supervisors: what social workers say they need to provide effective services. *British Journal of Social Work* **43** (8) 1562–1588.

Howard F, Beddoe L & Mowjood A (2013) Interprofessional supervision in social work and psychology in Aotearoa New Zealand. *Aotearoa New Zealand Social Work* **25** (4) 25–40.

Hudson B (2002) Interprofessionality in health and social care: the Achilles' heel of partnership? *Journal of Interprofessional Care* **16** (1) 7–17.

Hudson B (2007) Pessimism and optimism in inter-professional working: the Sedgefield Integrated Team. *Journal of Interprofessional Care* **21** (1) 3–15.

Hutchings J, Cooper L & O'Donoghue K (2014) Cross-disciplinary supervision amongst social workers in Aotearoa New Zealand. *Aotearoa New Zealand Social Work* **26** (4) 53–64.

McCallin A (2001) Interdisciplinary practice – a matter of teamwork: an integrated literature review. *Journal of Clinical Nursing* **10** (4) 419–428.

Mullarkey K, Keeley P & Playle JF (2001) Multiprofessional clinical supervision: challenges for mental health nurses. *Journal of Psychiatric and Mental Health Nursing* **8** (3) 205–211.

O'Donoghue K (2004) Social workers and cross-disciplinary supervision. *Social Work Review* **16** (3) 2–7.

Rains E (2007) Interdisciplinary supervisor development in a community health service. *Social Work Review* **19** (3) 58–65.

Scaife J (2009) *Supervision in Clinical Practice: A practitioner's guide* (2nd edition). London: Routledge.

Simmons H, Moroney H, Mace J & Shepherd K (2007) Supervision across disciplines: fact or fantasy In: D Wepa (Ed.) *Clinical Supervision in Aotearoa/New Zealand: A health perspective* (pp72–86). Auckland: Pearson Education.

Strong J, Kavanagh D, Wilson J, Spence SH, Worrall L & Crow N (2004) Supervision practice for allied health professionals within a large mental health service. *The Clinical Supervisor* **22** (1) 191–210.

Townend M (2005) IPS from the perspectives of both mental health nurses and other professionals in the field of cognitive behavioural psychotherapy. *Journal of Psychiatric & Mental Health Nursing* **12** (5) 582–588.

Chapter 5

Exploring service user involvement in adult health and social care supervision

Dr Tish Marrable and Sharon Lambley

The supervision that workers in social care and health services receive is generally agreed to be of great importance in supporting workers and providing good services to those they support. In its press release for new resources related to supervision, the Social Care Institute for Excellence (SCIE) stated that: *'Supervision is a vital skill to get right in social care and support services; the nature of the work can be emotionally charged and this can place particular demands on staff'* (SCIE, 2013). While what happens in supervision varies according to occupational focus and level of professional training of workers (Davys & Beddoe, 2010), in most areas of social and health care with adult service users it serves a number of purposes. It provides a place for staff management, for decision making about case management, for the development of the practitioner, as well as a space for the practitioner to reflect on their own involvement in the relationships that are part of service provision in adult social care services. One worker in our study described the complexity of the supervision process as 'interweaving', with each purpose feeding into the others in order to make the whole more than just the sum of its parts.

> *'But the whole thing interweaves the whole time, so from the supervisions I'm discussing my needs; I'm also discussing the needs of the service user and what I need to support him and how you can support me and how I can support you and the whole thing works that way.'*
> (Senior support worker, Lambley & Marrable, 2013)

Supervision has a long and respected place in practice, although it is not provided consistently (Care Quality Commission, 2013) and the reality of supervision does not always reflect the ideal of a regular, safe space for reflection, or well organised groups in a quiet space for discussion (Lambley & Marrable, 2013). Nor is a strong empirical evidence base available for the effectiveness of supervision (Carpenter *et al*, 2013) and what exists is mostly drawn from supervision studies within children and family services rather than from work with adults (Carpenter *et al*, 2012). Carpenter and colleagues state that: *'The overall aim of professional supervision should be to provide the best possible support to service users in accordance with the organisation's responsibilities and accountable professional standards'* (Carpenter *et al*, 2012 p3) but conclude from their review

of the literature that: *'no study reports on the perspectives of service users, hence the literature is silent on users' and carers' views on supervision.'*

In this chapter, we consider this missing element in supervision practice: the perspective and role of the service user. Our thinking about this arose from a practice enquiry we conducted for the SCIE which partnered with the Carpenter *et al* (2012) study. The study asked what good supervision practice looked like in adult services in England and Northern Ireland, where health and social care practitioners were working together (Lambley & Marrable, 2013). In order to gather evidence we spoke with workers and managers who identified good supervision practices in their workplace, and spoke separately to service users to ask them what their views were about professional supervision. Drawing on the study, this chapter first asks why service users should be involved in what has been seen as an element of support for workers, disconnected from the direct relationship of practice. It then considers the reasons that service users say that they should be involved in worker supervision and what they see as the issues. As a part of this, we will look at what service users can bring to supervision and provide some initial suggestions, drawn from both service user perspectives and those of workers, on how this might be done.

Introducing the study

The SCIE study was commissioned in 2011 as part of their work on developing a 'good practice framework'; in this case focusing on good practice in supervision in adult health and social care. SCIE wanted findings from at least three different types of practice, such as a community mental health team, a team supporting older people and a nursing or residential establishment. In order to find key sites, the University of Sussex team began the research with an online, mixed methods survey which gained 136 responses from workers in 28 different sites where staff perception was that good supervision was taking place. Participants were engaged in social work, in care roles, or health and well-being services such as nursing and therapeutic practices; just over half of them (51%) were supervisors as well as being supervised. Sites included local authority and NHS services, social enterprises, and for-profit providers. The survey was followed by four qualitative case studies drawn from the surveyed sites, chosen both for the reported strength of their supervision practices and to provide a fitting range of settings for these practices. While this did mean that there was no single model of good practice, it also let us look across the settings for elements that were common to all. The final stage to the data collection consisted of two focus groups with service users in order to gather their views on supervision in the services they received (Lambley & Marrable, 2013).

As researchers we believed that it was important to consider more than the supervisor/supervisee relationship when looking at 'good' supervision, since factors such as the work environment and protocol are influential, and the outcomes from supervision are not only for the individual worker, but also have an effect on the outcomes of those who use services and on the organisation as well (Lambley & Marrable, 2013). For this reason a systems approach (Reder *et al*, 1993; Fish *et al*, 2008) was taken throughout the research, looking at organisations and what goes on within them as a system for study. We used the organisational edges as a 'soft boundary' for the research since individual organisations are permeated by local and national policy and guidance on practice. We considered organisational structures as the conditions for supervision, the processes and practices within these, and the effects of these for stakeholders (Figure 5.1).

This approach was used in all parts of the data collection. For example, within each of the qualitative case studies, staff were asked about organisational resources, the supervision processes and outcomes from the supervision which they had judged as 'good', so as to gain a fuller picture of what made good supervision. A set of questions within the interviews asked for specific examples of better outcomes which arose from supervision for those using services, as well as for staff themselves and for the organisation.

While it was important to find out from practitioners about the outcomes of supervision for service users, an area where there is little strong evidence (Carpenter *et al*, 2013), it was equally important to gain the views of service users about supervision. Did they know about supervision, and what did they think was important about it? Was it clear to them what happened within supervision, and how it affected them and their relationships with workers? Did they have thoughts about what would constitute good practice? In order to find this out, we spoke with two service user groups, one made up of 11 people receiving services through community mental health (hereafter called focus group A), and the other a group of five adults with learning disability who formed an advisory group for their local Learning Disabilities Board (focus group B). Between them, these participants had experience of multiple health and social care professionals, management and care staff, housing and voluntary organisations. The findings from these groups were then presented to the SCIE advisory board for the study and a service user workshop at SCIE was convened to discuss and expand on the findings (Lambley *et al*, 2013).

Why should service users be involved in supervision?

For those adults who need health and social care services, having their wishes and views taken into account is an important part of receiving high quality services. Tambuyzer and Audenhove (2013, p675) argue that service user involvement in services has become a 'worldwide trend' emerging from the 1948 Universal Declaration of Human Rights and summarised in the phrase 'nothing about us without us'. This trend should not be seen as internationally or nationally uniform however. Service user organisations may have similar aims in prioritising the voices of those who use services, but emphasise this in different ways, reflecting a

Figure 5.1: Researching supervision using a systems approach (Lambley & Marrable, 2013)

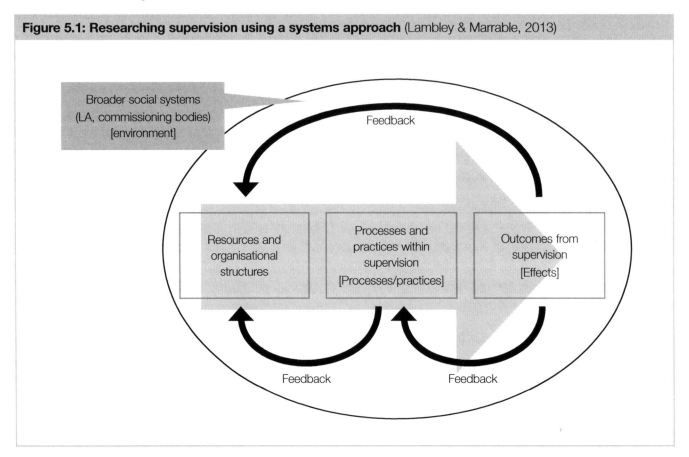

range of working relationships with organisations and services (Beresford & Branfield 2006). Services themselves also approach participation in different ways.

In England, recent guidance for the Care Act (2014) sets out service user involvement in decision making as one of the act's key principles, linking it to the personalisation agenda:

'…the importance of the individual participating as fully as possible in decisions about them and being provided with the information and support necessary to enable the individual to participate. Care and support should be personal, and local authorities should not make decisions from which the person is excluded.' (Department of Health, 2014, p4)

While a principle has no requirement for action attached, it sets a tone for services, a 'common expectation' that people who use services should be deeply involved in shaping their own care plans. How they are involved and what 'service user participation' (Department of Health, 2014) means in practice is not always clear however (McLaughlin, 2009; Tambuyzer *et al*, 2014). Simmons (2009) suggests that participation can take place in a number of ways depending on how the person is positioned by services, or positions themselves. For some, where decision making has been delegated to professionals, participation will be by proxy, and others will expect to speak for them, sometimes without consultation. The reluctant service user may be forced to use services and their participation can reflect this coercive relationship, while those who see themselves as customers may bring a different set of 'rational action' expectations with them; that choice, or purchase, produces good services. Finally, a model of collective participation sees the service user's voice feeding into the

co-production of service provision. These categories are fluid, so that the reluctant user might become a co-producer at a later point. To illustrate this, some members of focus group A in our study had experienced sectioning for mental health difficulties in the past, however they now positioned themselves as active co-producers of provision. Members of focus group B saw themselves as customers, and expected their voices and wishes to be heard as part of their active citizen's rights.

The way people using services are positioned is important in that it may alter the way that they contribute to decision making, either through their choice or through 'auto-exclusion' (Simmons, 2009) due to, for instance, a perceived lack of capacity. Nonetheless, if the Care Act's principle of participation in decision making is to be realised, then methods and spaces to do this must be found. Supervision is frequently used for decision making about provision, but service users have largely been excluded from this space.

To check supervision activity, the practice enquiry survey asked the worker participants what went on in their sessions, and whether it happened every time they had supervision, most of the time, occasionally or never. Two of these questions focused particularly on discussing service user cases and making decisions about the actions to take here (Figure 5.2).

In the first sub-question, *'Do you discuss progress for each service user/clients/cases'*, 75% of the sample (102 participants) replied, and from these, 75% (77) said they discussed this everytime, or most of the time. In the second, *'Do you make decisions about actions with service users/ clients/cases'*, the numbers were higher. 78% of the total sample responded (106 participants), and of these, 79% (89) made decisions about service users every time, or most of

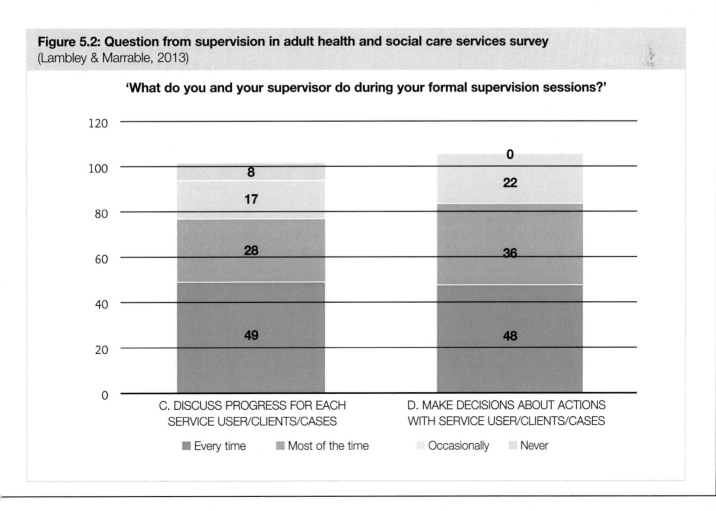

Figure 5.2: Question from supervision in adult health and social care services survey
(Lambley & Marrable, 2013)

'What do you and your supervisor do during your formal supervision sessions?'

the time. Out of those who answered this question, all used supervision as a place to make decisions about actions at least occasionally. This does not, however, suggest that each service user case was discussed, or had decisions made about it in each session, but highlights that supervision is a place in which this does occur.

The two service user focus groups within the study had clear views about why they should be involved, although different levels of knowledge about supervision itself. The consensus from focus group B was that, if staff were meeting and talking about them, they should be involved in this discussion. Only one of the group knew that staff had supervision, and this group member was only aware as they had been given a supervisor themselves when undertaking work experience. Despite seeing themselves as customers, they spoke of having little ability to influence their services and it often took a long while, and a great deal of persistence, for a request for change to be met. An example of this was where a group member had requested that they be provided with a female key worker, as there were issues with their care that they felt unable to discuss with their current male worker. They were told by a staff member that 'the service user couldn't choose' their keyworker. They next took this request to their care plan review meeting, but afterward felt 'told off' by the manager for raising this matter at this meeting, rather than before the meeting with the manager. They were given a new support worker four months after they had first made the request. Being involved in the staff member's supervision process would have allowed them to raise this matter at the point of decision making.

Within focus group A there was more awareness that supervision took place, as well as about the issues that affected their care such as heavy caseloads and a lack of resources. While they weren't sure what happened in the supervision process, they wanted to know how workers made sure that what service users want, think and feel is heard within it. They wanted to know how they could be more involved in supervision, as it was concerned with them and their care, but also understood that workers needed to have time with a supervisor to talk about their feelings because: 'they have to deal with some of our difficult feelings and it can be difficult for them'. However, they felt it was important to maintain a service user focus in supervision since it was their care or treatment that was in question. Like those in focus group B, many had experiences of difficulty in having their wishes heard. As one person said, 'you are told that you are in control but the reality is that you are not'. Involvement in worker supervision could provide a point of access into better 'control', whether through co-producing the service itself, or as customers, entitled to a good service which takes their choices into account.

What can service users bring to workers' supervision and how might they do this?

Pawson et al (2003), in their review of the kinds of knowledge that shape social care, identified service user knowledge as one of the five equally valuable sources for evidence, alongside policy, research, organisational and practice knowledge. Each kind of knowledge has its own purpose, and for service users this is to bring in their own expertise about their lives and experiences, as well as their perceptions of how services and helpers are functioning in providing care and support. As services move away from 'provider-centric' organisation into a consumer and co-produced paradigm (Bovaird, 2007; Simmons, 2009) the value of service user knowledge within supervision, in improving the quality of services for workers as well as their own support, needs to be more fully acknowledged.

The practice enquiry and the SCIE service user seminar provided some strong examples of different ways in which service users' input into supervision had made a difference within the service. On one level this input was able to forestall more serious consequences, as one participant stated in the SCIE seminar, 'things should not be allowed to fester until they become a complaint' (Lambley et al, 2013, p7). But service user input was also able to promote innovation within services, taking people's direct suggestions for improvements in their care and using the supervision process to work through how these could help to change practice overall. An example of this was in a residential home. A senior worker described how residents' meetings provided innovative ideas for improving services. These were brought into worker supervision and used as a way to support service user driven change. A study led by Shaping Our Lives, a service user led network which researches and promotes service user involvement, focused on what service users wanted from social care services for adults. Improving the quality of services was seen as a key role of service user involvement in services (Beresford et al, 2005), and the examples of innovating change provided here show that input into supervision could help to do this.

Within the online survey, worker participants spoke of the outcomes of supervision for service users in relation to their own well-being; a well-supported worker with space to reflect on their practice becomes more effective in their work. While this focused on the supervisor-supervisee relationship, it is helpful to consider how direct input from people using services can also provide support or implement positive change. Members of the service user focus groups were aware that workers often had caseloads that stretched their capability to the limit, and thought that one of the roles they could play in supervision was to speak up about this, essentially advocating for the worker's well-being. Workers also spoke of improvements in their well-being as a result of service users' views being considered in supervision. For example, one professionally qualified member of a community based team spoke about how service user feedback had helped them to improve their workload management and personal well-being. The worker had been suffering with migraines, which had caused them to cancel meetings with the service user. Feedback helped them to understand that continuity and reliability was important to the service user. They were able to work in their supervision to find ways to slow down, manage their health problems, and negotiate meeting less often with the service user, but becoming more reliable and available in other ways as a result of this.

For service users in the study, supervision was a key place for workers to discuss individuals' wishes related to service delivery. An example of this was where a resident with learning disabilities wanted to take part in a new gardening programme. The logistics of this were worked out in supervision with the result of a successful application to participate. Even where requests were not successfully fulfilled, if service users could see that workers had taken their wishes into account and done what they could within the resources available, they were satisfied. For example, a mental health service user had been offered cognitive behavioural therapy but didn't like the approach and wanted psychotherapy instead. Through discussion in supervision, it was agreed that the therapeutic route should be changed for the service user. However, there were no female psychotherapists available and this was an essential condition for this service user. Although disappointed, the service user accepted that workers had done their best, even if the service requested was not provided.

Although it was outside the scope of our study, the supervision of personal assistants (PAs) was a vital point for many service users. It was noted that funding was not available for PA supervision and this was a barrier for most of those employing them. A mother who was a social worker herself spoke about providing supervision for her daughter's PA and how this had helped to make her daughter's needs clear, and one PA at the SCIE seminar was able to speak about receiving supervision and how it had helped to build their knowledge for work (Lambley et al, 2013).

The examples above show that service user involvement in supervision already takes place in a number of ways, though when asked directly only one manager from the practice enquiry was able to say that this was part of their service delivery policy. While some participants in the focus groups expressed a wish to be actively involved in the supervision process itself, most sought less hands-on opportunities for their thoughts on service to be known. Forms, comment or feedback postcards directly to management, or questionnaires about care were generally favoured, but it was clear from poor experiences with complaint forms that management acknowledgment and follow-up were required for these to be seen as effective. Participants suggested that they could provide input into support plans which would be used in supervision to monitor progress alongside their wishes and to raise points to discuss with them. They emphasised that positive feedback about service provision was important to ensure that good practice was recognised and rewarded.

Complaints procedures were not seen as a good way for service users to feed into supervision; those that the focus groups had come across were not perceived as helpful. Participants wondered why supervisors didn't seem to know about poor services when complaints had been made, and why they didn't improve services when they did know. They expressed concern about complaining as they felt it could be unsafe for them, and they worried about repercussions from workers who were in powerful positions in relation to their support. However, it was noted within the service user seminar that the improved relationships that could arise from a stronger service user presence in professional processes had the potential to reduce complaints and work through issues before they became ingrained problems.

Conclusions

Listening to service users about their care is an essential part of providing good services, and finding ways to bring their thoughts, wishes and opinions directly into supervision can provide an effective way to do this. While it was clear in our study that people who use health and social care services see their relationship with organisations in different ways, both 'customers' and 'co-producers' wanted an active role if decisions were being made about their care and support. Service users could have a strong role in supervision through providing constructive feedback to workers so that they can challenge attitudes and practices that have become engrained; participants in both focus groups spoke of the negativity of some workers, of being seen as their diagnostic label rather than as a person and of being treated like children. Demonstrating respect and consideration for service users should be a primary goal in health and social care, and providers need to work with service users to ensure this happens. Beresford and Branfield wrote in 2006:

> 'Not engaging on full and equal terms with the end user raises moral and ethical issues, as well as creating practical difficulties for other partners, through failing to enable them to gain the benefits of service users' perspectives, experience, insights, ideas and knowledge. It creates a serious form of bias by omission.' (Beresford & Branfield, 2006, p443)

Involving service users in supervision may be uncomfortable for service providers to think about, however if the quality of services is to be improved and this moral issue, the 'bias by omission' is to be addressed, then ways must be found for this to be done.

References

Beresford P & Branfield F (2006) Developing inclusive partnerships: user-defined outcomes, networking and knowledge – a case study. *Health and Social Care in the Community* **14** (5) 436–444.

Beresford P, Shamash M, Forrest V, Turner, M & Branfield F (2005) *Developing Social Care: Service users' vision for adult support* [online]. London: Social Care Institute for Excellence in association with Shaping Our Lives. Available at: http://www.scie.org.uk/publications/reports/report07.asp (accessed November 2015).

Bovaird T (2007) Beyond engagement and participation: user and community coproduction of public services. *Public Administration Review* **65** (5) 846–650.

Care Quality Commission (2013) *The State of Health Care and Adult Social Care in England In 2012/13.* London: TSO.

Carpenter J, Webb C M, Bostock L, Coomber C (2012) *Effective Supervision in Social work and Social Care.* London: Social Care Institute for Excellence.

Carpenter J, Webb CM, Bostock L (2013) The surprisingly weak evidence base for supervision: findings from a systematic review of research in child welfare practice (2000-2012). *Children and Youth Services Review* **35** (11) 1843–1853.

Davys A & Beddoe L (2010) *Best Practice in Professional Supervision: A guide for the helping professions.* London: Jessica Kingsley

Publishers.

Department of Health (2014) *Care and Support Statutory Guidance Issued under the Care Act 2014*. Available at: https://www.gov.uk/government/publications/care-act-2014-statutory-guidance-for-implementation (accessed November 2015).

Fish S, Munro E, Bairstow S (2008) *Learning Together to Safeguard Children: Developing an inter-agency systems approach for case reviews*. London: Social Care Institute for Excellence.

Lambley S & Marrable T (2013) *Practice Enquiry into Supervision in a Variety of Adult Care Settings where there are Health and Social Care Practitioners Working Together*. London: Social Care Institute for Excellence.

Lambley S, Marrable T & SCIE (2013) *Service User and Carer Involvement in the Supervision of Health and Social Care Workers: Seminar Report*. London: Social Care Institute for Excellence.

McLaughlin H (2009) What's in a name: 'client', 'patient', 'customer', 'consumer', 'expert by experience', 'service user'—what's next? *British Journal of Social Work* **39** (6) 1101–1117.

Pawson R, Boaz A, Grayson L, Long A & Barnes C (2003) *Types and Quality of Knowledge in Social Care*. London: Social Care Institute for Excellence.

Reder P, Duncan S & Gray M (1993) *Beyond Blame: Child abuse tragedies revisited*. London: Routledge.

SCIE (2013) *Supervision in Social Care – New Resources from SCIE* [online]. SCIE press release. Available at: http://www.scie.org.uk/news/mediareleases/2013/220513.asp (accessed November 2015).

Simmons R (2009) Understanding the 'differentiated consumer' in public services. In: R Simmons, M Powell & Greener I (Eds) The *Consumer in Public Services Choice, Values and Difference*. Bristol: Policy Press.

Tambuyzer E, van Audenhove C (2013) Service user and family carer involvement in mental health care: divergent views. *Community Mental Health Journal* **49** (6) 675–685.

Tambuyzer E, Pieters G & van Audenhove C (2014) Patient involvement in mental health care: one size does not fit all. *Health Expectations: An International Journal of Public Participation in Health Care and Health Policy* **17** (1) 138–150.

Part II:

Innovations in practice: Models of supervision in a variety of settings

Introduction to Part II

Part II presents approaches to supervision that are established in their own professional setting, but may be novel and interesting to others. Some provide very clear models of supervision while others invite us to move beyond traditional forms of supervision and offer new ways of thinking and being, drawing on different disciplines and philosophies including mindfulness and coaching. All have a focus on supporting emotional well-being and understand that compassion in care can only be developed if professionals recognise, and feel supported to understand, their own vulnerabilities and how this can impact on service delivery.

In Chapter 6, Jane Wonnacott, director of In-Trac Training and Consultancy outlines a model of supervision first developed by the late Tony Morrison. The 4x4x4 model is an integrated framework that brings together the four functions, four stakeholders and four main processes involved in supervision. These elements have all been separately described in the literature, but the 4x4x4 model integrates them into a single model that can be used to underpin supervision practice in a variety of settings and contexts.

Following on from this, Sonya Wallbank, CEO of Capellas Group and consultant clinical psychologist, introduces her model of restorative resilience supervision in Chapter 7. First developed in response to the emotional demands of midwives, doctors and nurses caring for families who had experienced miscarriage and stillbirth, the model is designed to support the professionals to process their workplace experiences and support them to build resilience levels and coping strategies beyond the initial life of the supervision sessions. Sonya and Jane have been working together to introduce this model within the emotionally challenging context of safeguarding children's services.

In Chapter 8, Andy Bradley, founder of Frameworks 4 Change and one of Britain's top 50 radical thinkers as recognised by NESTA in conjunction with *The Observer* newspaper, explores the evolution of what he describes as compassion coaching. This approach emerged in response to his concerns that conventional models of supervision used in residential care homes were missing something – compassion. He provides us with a guide to compassion coaching that can be used in any setting or organisational context, supporting reciprocal and nurturing relationships to flourish.

Finally, Chapter 9 is co-authored by Rhiannon Barker and Esther Flanagan, programme managers with the Point of Care Foundation. Like Andy's chapter, they also reflect on how best to create conditions whereby practitioners are empowered to deliver compassionate care. They introduce us to Schwartz Rounds, developed in the US and initially used in healthcare settings, these reflective forums offer staff the space to discuss the social and emotional aspects of care with colleagues from across disciplines and positions, both clinical and non-clinical, whether doctors, nurses, social workers or hospital porters.

Chapter 6

A model for effective supervision in health and social care: Morrison's 4x4x4 model

Jane Wonnacott

This chapter outlines a model of supervision known as the 4x4x4 model which was first developed by Tony Morrison (2005) and used to deliver supervision training to a wide range of practitioners working in health and social care in the UK, Australia, New Zealand and Canada. In 2009, Morrison and In-Trac Training and Consultancy were commissioned to deliver a national training programme for the supervisors of newly qualified social workers and this provided the opportunity to test the approach and associated training materials with a large sample across England. An evaluation of the newly qualified social workers project included consideration of the impact of the 4x4x4 model and found that, where this had been fully implemented, stress was reduced and there were improvements in job satisfaction, worker retention and worker effectiveness (Carpenter *et al*, 2012).

The model has also been used to train supervisors working within interprofessional teams. It provides a common language for exploring the experience of the service user and the varying factors that may be affecting service delivery; including inter-professional communication and the differing values, attitudes and beliefs that practitioners bring to their work.

Following Tony Morrison's untimely death in 2010, the model has continued to evolve (Wonnacott, 2012; 2014) and form the foundation of training for supervisors across a range of health and social care organisations. This chapter draws on material already published by Pavilion (Morrison, 2005) with the intention of providing a summary of the model as well as consideration of where future developments might lie.

The core components of the 4x4x4 supervision model

Recognition that supervision makes a difference to outcomes for service users

This approach to supervision has at its heart a recognition that supervision is much more than a 'nice to have' added extra; it has a fundamental impact on the way staff feel about their work, their behaviour towards service users and colleagues and their knowledge and skills. As a result, supervision has a fundamental impact on the experience of service users and ultimately outcomes for adults, children and their families.

The importance of the supervisory relationship

This approach to supervision recognises the centrality of relationships and the importance of developing a positive relationship between the supervisor and the supervisee, which is then mirrored in the way that the supervisee works with service users. Positive relationships result in open, honest discussions where good practice can be celebrated and learnt from, and practice challenges, including mistakes, can be acknowledged and used as a vehicle to improve.

The role of the supervision agreement as a foundation for the relationship

Positive relationships will develop where the supervisor takes time to get to know the supervisee and where the boundaries and expectations of the supervisory process are clear, documented and regularly reviewed. Too often supervision contracts or agreements fail to take into account the individual nature of each supervisory relationship. Central to this model is the need to pay attention to all the factors that might impact on the relationship and to make sure that these are 'on the table' rather than 'under the table' where they could unintentionally inhibit open and honest exploration of relevant issues.

The interrelationship between feelings, thoughts and action

The 4x4x4 model stresses the importance of working with emotions, valuing intuitive responses and combining these with analytical thinking in order to inform judgements, decisions and plans. This is particularly important since:

'A system that seeks to ignore emotions is in danger of leaving them to have an unknown and possibly harmful impact on the work, and is also neglecting a rich source of data to help us understand what is going on.' (Munro, 2008)

The role of the supervision cycle in promoting reflective practice, critical thinking and defensible (recorded) decision making

At the heart of this approach is the supervision cycle. Based on Kolbs's (1984) adult learning cycle it encourages supervisors to ask questions which move beyond task completion to understanding the interrelationship between feelings, thoughts and actions. As such the model allows for an approach which recognises that often in the human services, decisions are based on professional judgement and are finely balanced. Recording the reasons for decisions becomes easier when supervision has allowed space for the critical reflection and critical thinking underpinning the work to take place.

An integrated approach to the delivery of supervision: the 4x4x4 model

Supervision has to address a range of requirements on behalf of different stakeholders, involving a complex set of activities. The 4x4x4 model is an integrated framework that brings together the functions, stakeholders and main processes involved in supervision. These elements have all been separately described in the literature, but the 4x4x4 model integrates them into a single model which can underpin supervision practice in a variety of settings and contexts.

The importance of the model is that it recognises the interdependence of the functions of supervision, their impact on key stakeholders and the supervision cycle as a process which ensures a focus on all the functions.

The 4x4x4 supervision model therefore brings together the:

→ four functions of supervision (management, development, support, mediation)

→ four key stakeholders in supervision (service users, staff, organisation, partners)

→ four elements of the supervisory cycle (experience, reflection, analysis, plans and actions).

The four functions of supervision

The early supervision literature (Kadushin, 1976) identified three main functions of supervision: management, support and development. Later, mediation was added (Richards et al, 1990) as the role of the supervisor at the interface of a number of different systems became understood. These functions are integral to the definition of supervision adapted by Morrison (2005) from the work of Harries (1987), namely:

'Supervision is a process by which one worker is given responsibility by the organisation to work with another worker(s) in order to meet certain organisational, professional and personal objectives which together promote the best outcomes for service users.

The four objectives or functions of supervision are:

→ *competent, accountable performance/practice (management function)*

→ *continuing professional development (development function)*

→ *personal support (support function)*

→ *engaging the individual with the organisation (mediation function).'*

(Morrison, 2005)

Within this definition it is important to consider the term 'management', since in some settings the main supervisory relationship is with someone other than the line manager. This may particularly be the case in interprofessional teams where, in order to ensure that practitioners receive supervision from within their own profession, supervision is provided by an experienced practitioner who has no direct line management responsibility for the supervisee. 'Management' is used broadly here to refer to the role that any supervisor has (whether or not they are the supervisee's line manager) in being accountable for any advice given and practice decisions that emerge from supervision. All supervisors will also have a responsibility to identify and report practice that might put a service user at risk.

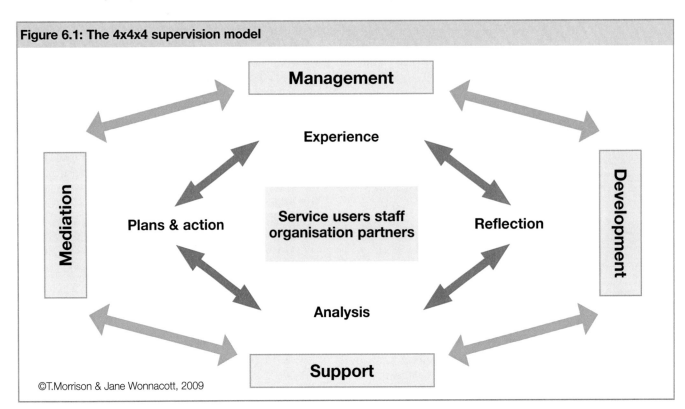

Figure 6.1: The 4x4x4 supervision model

Management

Experience

Mediation

Plans & action

Service users staff organisation partners

Reflection

Development

Analysis

Support

©T.Morrison & Jane Wonnacott, 2009

Figure 6.2: Benefits of effective supervision

Benefits for multidisciplinary working

→ Role clarity for the worker.
→ Identifying appropriate expectations for others.
→ Ensuring worker communicates with, and listens, to other agencies.
→ Preparing workers for multidisciplinary meetings.
→ Appreciation of different roles, challenging stereotyping.
→ Helps workers to interpret other agencies.
→ Assists in mediating conflicts with other agencies, or negotiating over resources.

Benefits for users

→ Worker clearer, more focused.
→ More observant of users' strengths, needs and risks.
→ More attentive to process and the users' feelings.
→ More aware of power issues.
→ More able to involve user.
→ More evidence-based assessment.
→ More consistent service.
→ Clearer plans.

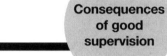

Consequences of good supervision

Benefits for the agency

→ Clearer communication both up and down.
→ Agency values and policies disseminated.
→ Increased sense of corporacy – working for the same organisation.
→ Improved standardisation.
→ Shared responsibility for problems.
→ Improved staff consultation processes.
→ Improved role understanding.
→ Greater openness.
→ Increased pride in the organisation.
→ Lower rates of turnover.

Benefits for staff

→ Role and accountability clear.
→ Work scrutinised.
→ Boundaries clarified.
→ Pressures shared.
→ Confidence enhanced.
→ Judgements reflected on.
→ Focus on user.
→ Creative practice supported.
→ Diversity valued.
→ Use/abuse of authority explored.
→ Poor practice challenged.
→ Learning needs identified.
→ Feelings addressed.
→ Worker valued, not isolated.
→ Team working enhanced.

Research has indicated that supervisors find it hard to pay equal attention to all four functions and that the management function may dominate (e.g. Gadsby Waters, 1992; Poertner & Rapp, 1983). Where any one function dominates it is problematic due to the interdependency of the four functions. For example, if it is clear that tasks are not being carried out then the supervisor will need to understand why. This may involve considering whether any factors such as stress or personal issues (support), lack of confidence or skill (development) or organisational factors (mediation) are affecting performance. In other instances (particularly in under-resourced teams where supervisors try to be a buffer between their staff and management demands), the support function may dominate, leading to a lack of challenge and poor performance.

The response to this tension has, in some organisations, been to separate the functions of supervision, with different supervisors being responsible for different aspects. For example, within health settings it is not unusual for a member of staff to receive separate clinical supervision in addition to separate managerial supervision and safeguarding supervision. The introduction of the restorative supervision model (Wallbank, 2013), which focuses on the emotional impact of the work and the development of worker resilience, is as a result of identifying the need to ensure that this aspect of supervision (support) is properly addressed.

The need to ensure that the emotional impact of the work is explored is particularly crucial in safeguarding work and a current development of the restorative and 4x4x4 models (Wallbank & Wonnacott, 2015) challenges the notion that

restorative supervision is a stand-alone supervisory process sitting outside of safeguarding supervision. They argue that effective safeguarding supervision needs to combine critical reflective practice and critical thinking with a restorative experience in order for the professional to feel supported and maintain their capacity to think.

Where a split approach is the preferred supervision system, attention needs to be paid to the totality of the supervisory experience of the supervisee and the risk of fragmentation and splitting between the supervisors. How will any concerns about the supervisee's practice that emerge in clinical or safeguarding supervision be addressed? How will the manager responsible for work allocation know about any personal factors or other stressors that should be taken into account? How will the roles and boundaries between the supervisors be established?

The four stakeholders in supervision

The second element of the 4x4x4 model focuses on the four main stakeholders, namely:

→ service users
→ supervisees
→ the organisation
→ partners, such as other organisations or professionals who also work with the same service users.

Figures 6.2 and 6.3 set out the consequences for the various stakeholders if the supervisory process is effective or ineffective.

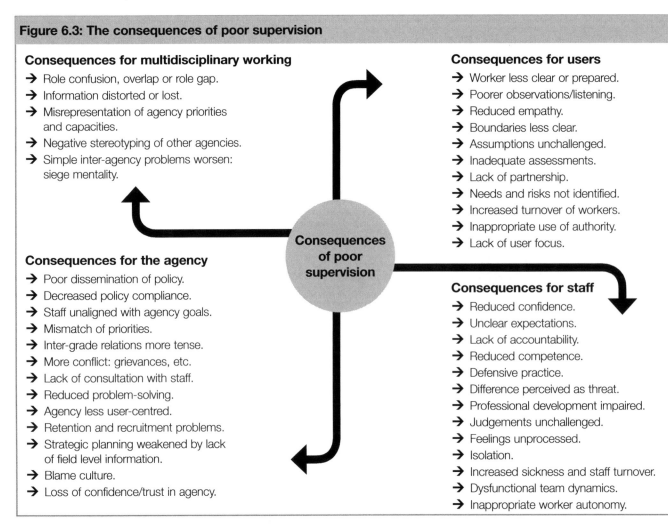

Figure 6.3: The consequences of poor supervision

Consequences for multidisciplinary working
→ Role confusion, overlap or role gap.
→ Information distorted or lost.
→ Misrepresentation of agency priorities and capacities.
→ Negative stereotyping of other agencies.
→ Simple inter-agency problems worsen: siege mentality.

Consequences for users
→ Worker less clear or prepared.
→ Poorer observations/listening.
→ Reduced empathy.
→ Boundaries less clear.
→ Assumptions unchallenged.
→ Inadequate assessments.
→ Lack of partnership.
→ Needs and risks not identified.
→ Increased turnover of workers.
→ Inappropriate use of authority.
→ Lack of user focus.

Consequences of poor supervision

Consequences for the agency
→ Poor dissemination of policy.
→ Decreased policy compliance.
→ Staff unaligned with agency goals.
→ Mismatch of priorities.
→ Inter-grade relations more tense.
→ More conflict: grievances, etc.
→ Lack of consultation with staff.
→ Reduced problem-solving.
→ Agency less user-centred.
→ Retention and recruitment problems.
→ Strategic planning weakened by lack of field level information.
→ Blame culture.
→ Loss of confidence/trust in agency.

Consequences for staff
→ Reduced confidence.
→ Unclear expectations.
→ Lack of accountability.
→ Reduced competence.
→ Defensive practice.
→ Difference perceived as threat.
→ Professional development impaired.
→ Judgements unchallenged.
→ Feelings unprocessed.
→ Isolation.
→ Increased sickness and staff turnover.
→ Dysfunctional team dynamics.
→ Inappropriate worker autonomy.

The key here is that while there may only be two stakeholders physically present in supervision (the supervisor and supervisee), almost invariably other stakeholders are also involved and affected by what happens in supervision. Therefore, this model stresses that an important task for the supervisor is to ensure that other stakeholders are kept in mind and engaged within the process.

The supervision cycle

This is the third element of the 4x4x4 model and focuses on the process of supervision itself, and its relationship with practice. The problem solving supervision diagram in figure 6.4 is actually made up of two cycles: the 'story' or practice cycle and the supervision cycle of experience, reflection, analysis and planning.

These parallel cycles describe the process of effective practice with service users and effective supervision, and show how they are intimately related.

The 'story' or practice cycle

This cycle shows that good practice in any setting occurs when the worker:

→ engages with the service user and their story and identifies the stories of other people who are involved
→ helps the user to identify the feelings generated by the story, and the feelings of others involved
→ helps the user to consider the meaning of the story, its causes, consequences and impact

→ helps the user to think about how they would like the next chapter of the story to be written, and what help they need to move the story on.

The supervision cycle as a model for reflective supervision

The same four stages of the cycle can be applied to the supervision process. The way in which the supervisor asks questions is as important as the way the worker elicits the user's story. Open-ended questions about the user and the context will generate a very different account of what happened than closed questions with a narrow focus. In other words, the worker's account and focus are shaped significantly by the questions asked by the supervisor.

Experience of training supervisors over a number of years has shown that developing skills in asking open questions needs constant reinforcement especially at times of stress or anxiety.

Experiencing

The origins of the supervision cycle lie in a theory of adult learning. According to Kolb (1984), learning is triggered by experience, either in terms of a problem to be solved, a situation that is unfamiliar, or a need that must be satisfied. Learning involves transforming experience into feelings (reflection), knowledge, attitudes and values (analysis), behaviours and skills (plans and action).

In professional terms, the cycle is triggered when the worker experiences a problem when undertaking a practice task, or when they identify a need such as practice development.

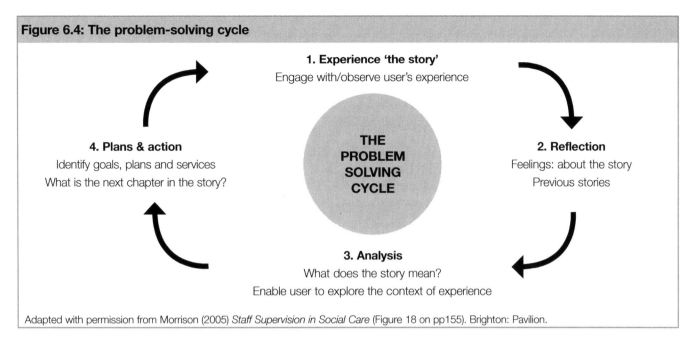

Figure 6.4: The problem-solving cycle

1. Experience 'the story'
Engage with/observe user's experience

THE PROBLEM SOLVING CYCLE

4. Plans & action
Identify goals, plans and services
What is the next chapter in the story?

2. Reflection
Feelings: about the story
Previous stories

3. Analysis
What does the story mean?
Enable user to explore the context of experience

Adapted with permission from Morrison (2005) *Staff Supervision in Social Care* (Figure 18 on pp155). Brighton: Pavilion.

Alternatively, the supervisor may trigger the cycle by asking the worker to review a case, or by seeking improved performance.

To make use of experience and to learn from it, there first has to be an engagement in that experience. For instance, the worker may complete the task while being psychologically disengaged with it. At this stage of the cycle, the task for the supervisor is to help the worker obtain accurate observations of what went on, and the nature of the user's circumstances. It cannot be assumed that, because the worker was present, accurate observations were made. Nor can it be assumed that in a busy office, when the supervisor asks 'What happened?' this will elicit a full account of the worker's observations. Instead, 'What happened?' may be shorthand for 'I only want to address urgent or high-risk matters, or offer immediate guidance.'

The account of practice comes as a result of the dialogue between supervisee and supervisor, and is significantly influenced by the ways in which the supervisor conducts that discussion and by the types of questions asked. Therefore, the practice cycle does not exist as an objective piece of information. Rather, the way in which the supervisor asks about the worker's observations shapes both the focus and scope of the practice account.

Reflecting

Engaging in experience is not sufficient. Without reflecting on the experience, it may be lost or misunderstood. For instance, the worker may have been engaged in a powerful piece of work but if the experience is not de-briefed or reflected on, its benefit may be lost or misunderstood.

Processing feelings often reveals a richer layer of observations, for example, observations held at an emotional level. Reflection explores feelings, patterns and connections arising from the experience. It is also through emotion that workers identify what values or assumptions are triggered by a piece of work.

The nature of the social care task can produce strong emotional and moral responses that need to be acknowledged and processed. It is also important to clarify the source of these responses. Sometimes we feel before

we see. For instance, gut reactions or feelings that can't be initially rationalised are sometimes clues to vital information about unspoken situations or dangers. When these are explored in supervision, the unconscious observations that resulted in these reactions can be uncovered.

For workers facing new demands and levels of responsibility, the opportunity to talk about the emotional demands of the work is particularly important and it is crucial that they receive the positive message that talking about emotions is a sign of strength and competence.

Analysis

Reflection should lead to analysis. If the cycle stops at reflection, false and subjective conclusions may be drawn. Analysis ensures that evidence and feelings are located within an external body of knowledge, theory, research and professional value, and then tested against it. Analysis translates information and observations into professional evidence. This occurs through interrogating information and probing discrepancies so that its meaning and significance can be elicited. It is how workers make sense of the situation and of their own assessment, intentions and plans. In doing so, analysis must incorporate the meaning of the situation to the user, as well as to the worker or their organisation. Analysis is essential in explaining and justifying intervention in people's lives, advocating resources or seeking external authority for action.

From a development perspective, analysis provides the basis for wider learning through generalisations that can be made from analysis done on a specific case. If this analysis is not done, and the worker moves straight from reflection to action, it is possible to get it 'right' without knowing why. Equally, if no analysis is done and things go wrong, it is impossible to understand why. This will prevent workers from being able to learn from difficulties or to improve their practice.

Action planning

In order to deliver effective services, the analysis needs to be translated into plans and actions. At this stage in the supervision cycle, the focus is on the planning, preparation and rehearsal of strategies.

Goals need to be set and practical options examined. Before the worker tries out a new approach or a change of tack, the supervisor may need to go through the plan with them, facilitate co-working or identify contingency plans. The supervisor's skills are important here, helping to generate and test different options. Finally, as strategies are put into action, the cycle moves into its next phase as new experience is created and a fresh cycle begins.

Avoiding short circuits and quick fixes

The supervision process can therefore be seen as a continuous cycle of experience, reflection, analysis, planning, action and review. For problem solving or development to be fully effective, all four parts of the learning cycle need to be addressed. The challenge for supervisors is to resist the temptation and/or pressure to move rapidly from experience to plan, with little or no focus on reflection and analysis. This is the 'short circuit'. As shown in figure 6.5: The quick fix, rushing or skipping the reflective and analytical stages of this process, might provide a quick fix solution, but also increases the likelihood of the problem recurring as it has not been sufficiently addressed.

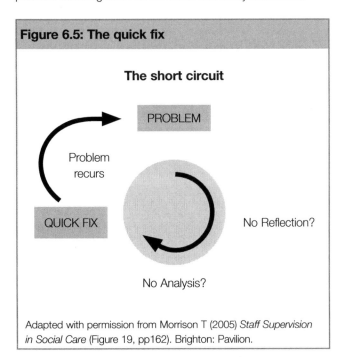

Figure 6.5: The quick fix

The short circuit

PROBLEM

Problem recurs

QUICK FIX

No Reflection?

No Analysis?

Adapted with permission from Morrison T (2005) *Staff Supervision in Social Care* (Figure 19, pp162). Brighton: Pavilion.

In addition, workers have different styles and preferences, so that while one social worker may engage easily in questions about feelings, another will find this much harder. Factors such as the practitioner's level of professional development, discipline, role, gender, language and class all contribute to their problem-solving style.

The model in the future

This model of supervision has stood the test of time and reports from trainers using this approach to develop supervision within health and social care in the UK continue to emphasise its relevance. In addition, it is particularly striking that reviews of practice continue to emphasise the importance of a style of supervision that helps practitioners to grapple with the complexity of their work and integrate both their intrusive responses with a reasoned analytical approach to decision making. Court judgements in child care cases stress the needs for improved analysis (Munby, 2015) yet the current climate for

health and social care in England is one where practitioners are increasingly required to make decisions in high stress environments while managing increased workloads. This model has much to offer in this environment because of the model's emphasis on developing resilient workers through a focus on the whole person, acknowledging the emotional impact of the work and challenging the worker to think differently, creatively and analytically about their practice. The integration of the 4x4x4 model with restorative supervision (see chapter 7 in this volume) may go some way to taking the model forward, while further work needs to be done to develop tools and approaches which support the use of the model in high stress, low resource environments (Wallbank & Wonnacott, 2015).

As practice in health and social care continues to evolve with a greater emphasis on working within interprofessional settings, this model needs to build on its core set of beliefs and values underpinning effective supervision and develop flexible tools and approaches. This has the potential to provide a common language for practitioners to reflect on both their own practice and those relationships across systems that have a significant impact on the day-to-day experience of service users.

References

Carpenter J, Patsios D, Wood M, Platt D, Shardlow S, Scholar H, Haines C, Wong C & Blewett J (2012) *Newly Qualified Social Worker Programme Final Evaluation Report* (2008-2011) Department of Education Research Report RR229.

Gadsby Waters J (1992) *The Supervision of Child Protection Work.* Aldershot: Avebury.

Harries (1987) *Discussion Paper on Social Work Supervision.* W. A. Branch of Australian Association for Social Workers.

Kadushin A (1976) *Supervision in Social Work.* New York: Columbia University Press.

Kolb D (1984) *Experiential Learning: Experience as a source of learning and development.* London: Prentice-Hall.

Morrison T (2005) *Staff Supervision in Social Care* (3rd edition). Brighton: Pavilion.

Munby (2015) EWFC 11: Case number MB14C01592.

Munro E (2008) *Effective Child Protection.* London: SAGE Publications Ltd.

Poertner J & Rapp CA (1983) What is social work supervision? *The Clinical Supervisor* **1** (2) 53–65.

Richards M, Payne C & Sheppard A (1990) *Staff Supervision in Child Protection Work.* London: National Institute of Social Work.

Wallbank S (2013) Recognising stressors and using restorative supervision to support a healthier maternity workforce: a retrospective, cross-sectional, questionnaire survey. *Evidence Based Midwifery* **11** (1) 4–9.

Wallbank S & Wonnacott J (2015) The integrated model of restorative supervision for use within safeguarding. *Community Practitioner*, **88** (5) 41–5.

Wonnacott J (2012) *Mastering Social Work Supervision.* London: JKP.

Wonnacott J (2014) *Developing and Supporting Effective Staff Supervision.* Brighton: Pavilion.

Chapter 7

Using restorative resilience supervision to support professionals to thrive

Dr Sonya Wallbank

'My mission in life is not merely to survive, but to thrive; and to do so with some passion, some compassion, some humor, and some style.'

Maya Angelou

The erosion of resilience

The focus of this paper is on information that will be useful to you in understanding why restorative resilience supervision has a positive impact on those professionals who undertake it. It is not designed to be an exhaustive review of the literature in areas such as stress, burnout and clinical supervision, but more a practical review of the model itself and why professionals have found it useful. Worker stress, burnout and lack of compassion appear to be a frequently reported theme associated with the helping professions. If you spend any amount of time with professionals working within the public and voluntary sectors they will describe the daily pressures that these environments are under. Budgetary restraints, increased public demand for services, as well as the changing population demographics mean that those working within the helping professions have a heightened vulnerability to stressors. The challenging working environment appears to foster within its workers a resigned acceptance that struggling to manage work demands is an integral part of this work:

'HSE says workers in health and social care have some of the highest rates of self-reported illness due to stress, anxiety and depression.' (NHS Employers, 2009, p1)

Given the cost to the public purse, with £300-400 million currently being spent in the NHS alone on sickness pay (NHS Employers, 2009), there is much incentive for organisations to get this right. As well as sickness absence, workers are also more likely to experience 'presenteeism'; where they feel unwell and should really be at home (Rayson, 2011). The way in which staff are feeling can result in an increase in accidents, errors, low morale, poor performance and can also have a significant impact on well-being, productivity and effectiveness (NHS Employers, 2009).

The impact of the environment on the worker is revealed in serious case reviews where competent, well trained professionals have demonstrated a reduced capacity to think. This often ends in tragic consequences and stretches beyond professional boundaries.

'Missed opportunities to protect Daniel and potentially uncover the abuse he was suffering occurred... In this case professionals needed to 'think the unthinkable...' (Coventry LSCB, 2013, p6)

'...there are places where unhealthy cultures, poor leadership and an acceptance of poor standards are too prevalent.' (Francis, 2013, p25)

While in the event of such tragedies, the dominant narrative focuses on the failings of the professionals, what seems to be missing is any understanding of why these things happen. Why do we assume that undertaking clinically complex work does not leave its mark on the professional? Why do highly trained professionals miss critical information, accept versions of events that do not correlate with evidence in front of them or make no sense, and have a reduced capacity to think and challenge? Why are we not ensuring robust support systems which improve and maintain the professionals' capacity to think?

Professional vulnerability

In order to remain emotionally well and engaged in work, professionals need to understand their own vulnerability and triggers and have a robust method of managing the impact of their work. The psychological responses or reactions of professionals working in the helping or caring professions have been the subject of many research papers. It is important to consider that while there are professionals who will exhibit severe reactions to their work context, the negative impact of the work environment is not necessarily obvious in others. Often professionals attracted to this type of work are coping with their everyday context by struggling quietly and will be displaying less obvious symptoms. This is partly due to the personality factors that are intrinsic to professionals who want to help and care for others; they are carers but can find it more challenging to recognise that they also need to be cared for.

The context in which these professionals work can also expect a high level of functional behaviour, focusing on the work at hand rather than thinking more deeply about it. This is perhaps why individual needs are not recognised because of the sheer demand of the work. This can make it difficult for those professionals to communicate, 'I need something for me', even where the work demands that the professional consistently gives of themselves. Occupational health serves to address the needs of the professional who is simply not coping, but this can be disingenuous to the professional. Being referred to occupational health means that this reaction is considered an individual problem rather than a naturally occurring reaction to the work context or content.

Vulnerability factors

1. Recognised vulnerability factors (Firth-Cozens, 1999) within the helping and caring workforce include the **level of commitment** individuals have to their jobs. This makes it difficult for the individual to operate in a boundaried way, instead opting to say yes to all that is asked of them.

2. **Job security**, or the lack of it, also means the professional becomes vulnerable to stressors. Given the level of change in a number of our public sector bodies, this must be a constant challenge.

3. **Unclear or conflicted expectations** are also a factor. This is a key feature of working in a multidisciplinary team, but the professional needs to have the presence of mind to be constantly renegotiating their role in relation to the wider team.

4. Working in a **hostile or defensive atmosphere** also increases vulnerability. We know that difficult behaviours increase as stress rises, so you are more likely to experience a challenging environment where demands are high.

5. Working in **an unethical environment** is a further risk to vulnerability. Individuals tend to be drawn into this work because of their personal values and the context that does not support that will compromise the individual.

6. Finally, a **lack of communication** increases risk. This is often a result of the pace of change meaning the level of communication cannot keep up.

Why restorative resilience supervision?

'... managers must recognise anxiety undermines good practice. Staff supervision and the assurance of good practice must become elementary requirements in each service.' (Department for Education, 2009, p7)

The model of restorative resilience supervision was first developed in response to the emotional demands of midwives, doctors and nurses caring for families who had experienced miscarriage and stillbirth (Wallbank, 2010). The programme was designed to support the professionals to process their workplace experiences and support them to build resilience levels to ensure they had future coping strategies beyond the initial life of the supervision sessions. The impact of the sessions on the professionals' levels

of stress, burnout and compassion satisfaction (pleasure derived from doing their job) was measured using The Professional Quality of Life Scale (Stamm, 2009). Results showed that after six sessions, compassion satisfaction was improved, while stress and burnout was reduced by over 40%.

Since the initial studies, the programme has been delivered to over 4,500 professionals (www.restorativesupervision.org. uk). The model of training has evolved from the sessions being delivered directly by a clinical psychologist to a range of professionals being trained to deliver the sessions themselves. This provides a sustainable model and ensures that the supervision can continue beyond the initial training sessions. The training model consists of a training day, no more than six sessions of individual supervision, followed by moving into small group supervision. The move into group supervision takes place to enhance the teamwork capacity of the supervisees and only once they are in a resilient enough state of mind for this experience to work well for them. The ongoing effectiveness of group supervision following the individual sessions has also been tested, showing not only how it maintains resilience, but also enhances workplace functioning (Wallbank, 2013). Access to further limited individual supervision is always kept open if a specific event or circumstance arises. Results continue to be consistent with reductions in stress and burnout and increases in compassion satisfaction (Wallbank, 2015).

Organisations implementing the restorative resilience model have conducted their own satisfaction surveys with patients and families in their care to review pre- and post-supervision data. The benefits of the supervision model have also moved beyond the supervisors themselves, with higher levels of patient and family satisfaction reported where staff were undertaking supervision (Department of Health, 2013). Staff also reported higher levels of satisfaction themselves with the care and interventions they were able to offer. Compassionate care experiences were also more evident (Wallbank, 2015).

Organisational impact has also continued to be measured where the programme has been cascaded. Inappropriate workplace behaviours are more likely to be challenged where the model of supervision has been implemented. Organisational attachment (St. Clair, 2000) also improves; this is the way in which individuals identify and work collaboratively with their employers. Sickness levels and turnover of staff decreases and the capacity of the professional to engage with others improves. An inadvertent benefit also appears to be the capacity the professional has to think about their own health behaviours. This meant they would talk about giving up smoking, losing weight or eating healthier. The sessions appeared to improve the capacity of the professional to think about themselves and their own attitude to health behaviours. This appeared to be as a result of the capacity of the professional to slow down their thinking and improve their decision making. Ultimately, the sessions ensured professionals were more effective in their work, able to demonstrate their boundaries and were calmer as a result (Wallbank, 2010).

'Ultimately, I feel stronger and I have greater thinking capacity... I also feel valued by my employer for recognising that this is a challenging time...' (Trueland, 2013)

What is the model?

Key principles

The training programme is built on a number of key principles which differ from usual models of supervision. Firstly, the supervision is person, and not case based. This enables the learning that the professionals takes from the supervision to be applied across their cases and is not just limited to the individual case discussion. We know from a range of serious case reviews that the capacity to implement learning across cases remains problematic (Wallbank & Wonnacott, 2015).

The time spent within the supervision session has to be effective for both the individual and the organisation. This is achieved by sharing sessions that are both negotiated and remain continuously relevant to both parties. The research around clinical supervision models demonstrates that too often supervisors are being asked to deliver supervision with little knowledge, skill or training and subsequently hours are spent in an ineffective cycle. Effective supervision can be used as a tool to bring organisations and individuals more closely aligned (Wallbank, 2015).

The importance of the context in which the professional works cannot be underestimated. Continuing to ensure that confidentiality is protected, feedback on the themes from supervision enables organisations to learn what needs to be changed or resolved quickly. Too often, the activity of supervision is entirely removed from the context in which it is taking place, decreasing its relevance to both the organisation and individual.

Finally, the process is not one of counselling or passive acceptance of information from the professional. Rather it reflects the need to challenge and engage with the professional to ensure that their resilience is improved. This requires supervisors to have engagement skills with their supervisees which enable them to deliver direct feedback supportively.

Supervisor's skills developed

The model of restorative resilience supervision draws on six key skills:

1. Emotional containment.
2. Reflective practice.
3. Stress inoculation.
4. Resilience training.
5. Action learning.
6. Foundation coaching.

The timeliness of intervention with each skill will depend upon where the supervisee is in terms of their own resilience and capacity to think. This is illustrated in figure 7.1.

Delivering supervision to a large number of professionals has shown us that the cognitive (thinking) approach and psychological state of the supervisee all influence their needs in supervision. We have developed 'zones' to describe the predominant states that supervisees seem to come into supervision sessions with and described some of the skills that you will need to support supervisees in these zones. This is not to suggest that the professional is only in one zone all the time, but it is the amount of time they spend there that influences their overall productivity.

Figure 7.1: Process of restorative resilience supervision (Wallbank, 2015)

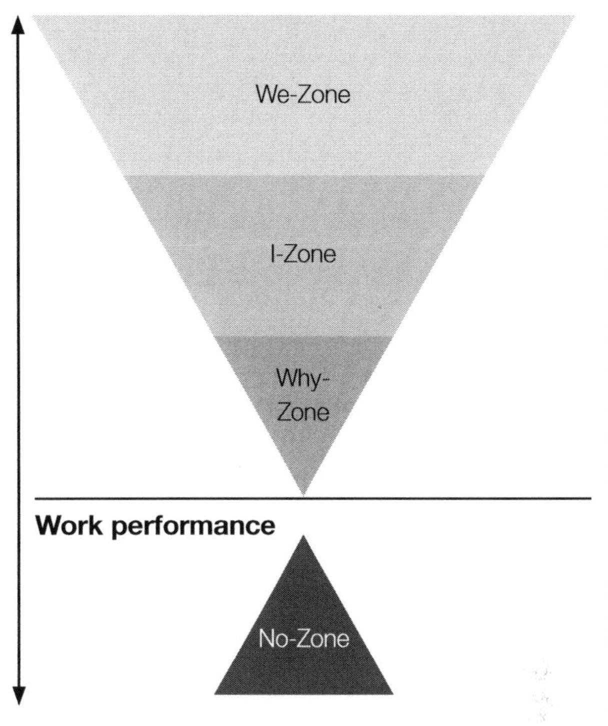

No-Zone

The professional who spends the majority of their time in this zone is usually one who is suffering the adverse effects of stress. They can be unnecessarily difficult or disruptive, or completely withdrawn/disengaged from the working environment. Energy levels for this professional would usually be low and you would recognise them as being quite difficult to sit with or talk to; often they feel slowed down or just difficult. They are more likely to be describing conflicts with others, whether this be other professionals, managers or people they are working with.

Why-Zone

This zone describes another more negative experience but it is a step up from the no-zone. Professionals are anxious and operate in a 'questioning everything' mode. This does not mean seeking useful information or clarification, but a nervous or fearful energy. There is often too much on their mind. Productivity is negative or neutral at best in this zone.

Professionals in the 'why-zone' are often consumed with an event or events that have taken place in the workplace. It could be a team dispute, difficult work experience where things did not go to plan, conflict or lack of progression. The important thing to bear in mind is that we will all experience being in this zone at some point. Our thinking skills are not great in this zone as we give all of our cognitive efforts to focusing on previous events which we are unable to change.

Both these zones require emotional containment, good listening skills and reflection to move professionals into a more positive place. Action learning sets and stress inoculation/resilience building (key tools to build on individuals' usual coping methods and areas of strength) ensure they do not go back down into these zones without strategies for exiting. It is the sense of being 'stuck' in the zone that causes problems. Functional professionals who learn skills to exit the areas still visit these zones but can equally leave them. The specific skills will be looked at in more detail later.

I-Zone

This is an energetic zone and tends to increase productivity. The professional is able to focus more on what they need to do to enhance their learning, practice or overall health and well-being. The talk in this zone is about what 'I' can do to learn, change or move my situation. The professional recognises their own behaviour and contribution to events/situations. They are thinking and expressing themselves clearly.

We-Zone

This is again a high energy area. The professional is creative and energetic, thinking of new ideas to benefit themselves, clients/patients and organisations. They are a pleasure to work around and you are energised from being with them. The discussions tend to be about the supervisee and others and their plans, and tend to be forward as well as outward-looking from their own job role and organisation.

In these zones we utilise coaching and action learning interventions including role playing with the more energetic zones. The idea is to ensure that you reflect back to the supervisee what the content of the conversations are, and what their positive triggers seem to be, so that they can begin to recognise this in themselves. This will help them identify what can interfere with their effectiveness, how they can support their own learning and growth and what their risk factors are.

Reflective practice is a key skill and will underpin all the zones as it ensures that emotive, difficult and frequent challenges can be learnt from.

Case example:

Deborah is a senior leader in a child and health family service and has over 20 years' experience in this work. The organisation she worked in had recently changed and the expectations of the new management were high. The increased demand of her role as well as the complexity of the work had left her with an overwhelming anxiety that she was not good enough and would be found out at any moment. Known within her workplace for 'putting a brave face on it', she was reluctant to let anyone know the extent of her anxiety. The supervisor worked with Deborah to enable her to reflect and process her experiences to get to the heart of what her actual concerns were. By reflecting back some of the self-deprecating comments that Deborah was making, they discussed why this was not useful as a senior leader who needed to portray confidence and gain respect. It transpired through the sessions that the lack of formal education Deborah had was a source of anxiety. Together they drew up a plan about how she could accredit the workplace experiences she had and move towards gaining a master's degree. Deborah's presentation changed through the sessions, becoming much less anxious and more able to think clearly. This enabled the supervisor to build a plan with her about moving the situation forward and reducing her anxiety in the future.

Recognising resilience

There are a number of key indicators that suggest the professional is demonstrating their capacity to remain resilient, and the objective of the sessions is therefore to work on improving the frequency of these.

→ Emotional intelligence – they are able to connect with others but not be overwhelmed by their experiences.

→ Able to deal with change – positive and negative narrative is balanced.

→ Positively engaged with their workplace.

→ High expectations of themselves and others.

→ Measured behaviours – not vulnerable to continuous highs and lows.

→ Clear and open communications.

→ Demonstrate problem solving skills.

→ Positive relationships with others.

→ Positive narrative relating to work – versus the 'them' and 'us' discussion.

→ Ability to utilise rules and consequences – knowing which ones to challenge.

→ Aspirational for their clients, self and/or organisation.

→ Boundaried behaviour – volunteers but able to express choice and control.

Case example:

Linda was a very experienced social worker and recognised as a source of knowledge and expertise. Consistent changes within the team structure and an endless supply of work had left Linda, by her own admission, with nothing left to give. Receiving restorative resilience sessions enabled Linda to focus on what was in her control to be able to change and what she needed to accept as a cost of doing the work. Linda became visibly more hopeful and energetic as the sessions continued, partly as she was able to let go of feeling the need to take responsibility for everything. Linda's team manager commented to the supervisor how much more engaged Linda had become and that for the first time since she could remember, Linda felt able to volunteer for a task during a meeting. The team around her had also commented on the difference, and that Linda was talking about work in a more positive light.

Universal lessons from using the approach

Organisations have the capacity to both mediate and exacerbate the vulnerability of their workforce to stress. By remaining in tune with the needs of the workforce and the specific demands of the role professionals are carrying out, their ability to remain resilient in the face of increasing demands will be improved. This will also ensure that programmes designed to support the needs of staff reflect their vulnerabilities rather than waiting until they have fallen over before the intervention is offered.

Training in supervision approaches is paramount if professionals are going to use this valuable time to benefit both them and their organisations. The quality and effectiveness of the supervision space is hugely varied, and the consistent narrative that supervision efficacy cannot be measured enables it to remain cloaked in mystery at best, in inadequacy at worst.

Recognising the need for professionals to work in a supportive environment is critical, especially where we are asking them to give of themselves. Inadvertent consequences of mobile working and open plan offices is the lack of individual contact between people. This means the low-level emotional support colleagues used to give each other has been compromised, making them more vulnerable to stress.

Professionals have a responsibility to understand how to prevent, minimise or overcome the potentially damaging effects of adversity through their work. Working with a lack of boundaries or continuing to give to the role beyond a physically or psychologically safe point is a responsibility shared between organisations and professionals. Recognising this and taking personal responsibility for the way in which we work needs to be the response of all professionals, rather than just continuing to protest that the role requires too much of them. Supporting newly qualified professionals to manage their work/life balance would seem to be an excellent start to working in a more boundaried way.

The model's utility seems appropriate across settings and workplaces, as the content of the model is the individual professional, not a specific client base. This also means that whether you are having direct client or patient access or have supervisory responsibilities, the tools used are the same. The learning, reflection and development that the supervisee engages in during the sessions can be applied across their case load or their management responsibilities.

References

Coventry LSCB (2013) *Final Overview Report of the Serious Case Review Re: Daniel Pelka* [online]. Available at: http://www.lgiu.org.uk/wp-content/uploads/2013/10/Daniel-Pelka-Serious-Case-Review-Coventry-LSCB.pdf (accessed November 2015).

Department for Education (2009) *The Protection of Children in England: A progress report* [online]. The Stationary Office, London. Available at: https://www.gov.uk/government/uploads/system/uploads/attachment_data/file/328117/The_Protection_of_Children_in_England.pdf (accessed November 2015).

Department of Health (2013) *Using Restorative Supervision to Improve Clinical Practice and Safeguarding Decisions* [online]. Available at: https://www.gov.uk/government/uploads/system/uploads/attachment_data/file/209911/S15_Restorative_Supervision_Surrey_EISCS_V121211.pdf (accessed November 2015).

Firth-Cozens J & Payne R (1999) *Stress in Health Professionals: Psychological and organisational causes and interventions*. Chichester: Wiley-Blackwell.

Francis R (2013) *Report of the Mid Staffordshire NHS Foundation Trust Public Enquiry* [online]. Available at: https://www.gov.uk/government/uploads/system/uploads/attachment_data/file/279124/0947.pdf (accessed November 2015).

NHS Employers (2009) *Stress Management* [online]. Available at: http://www.nhsemployers.org/~/media/Employers/Publications/Stress%20management.pdf (accessed November 2015).

Rayson M (2011) *How public sector sickness figures can aid a balanced debate about staff* [online]. The Guardian 8 August. Available at: http://www.theguardian.com/public-leaders-network/2011/aug/08/public-sector-sickness-figures-debate (accessed November 2015).

St. Clair L (2000) *Exploring the Psychodynamics of the employee relationship* [online]. Bryant College Faculty Working Paper Series. Available at: http://digitalcommons.bryant.edu/managework/1/ (accessed November 2015).

Stamm BH (2009) *The Concise PROQOL Manual*. Pocatello, Idaho: The ProQOL.org.

Trueland J (2013) Breathe new life into your flagging career. *Nursing Standard* **27** (37) 20–22.

Wallbank S (2010) Effectiveness of individual clinical supervision for midwives and doctors in stress reduction: findings from a pilot study. *Evidence Based Midwifery* **8** 65–70.

Wallbank S (2013) Maintaining professional resilience through group supervision. *Community Practitioner* **86** (8) 23–25.

Wallbank S (2015) *Restorative Resilience through Supervision*. Brighton: Pavilion. In press.

Wallbank S & Wonnacott J (2015) The integrated model of restorative supervision for use within safeguarding. *Community Practitioner* **88** (5) 41–5.

Wallbank S & Woods G (2012) A healthier health visiting workforce: findings from the Restorative Supervision Programme. *Community Practitioner* **85** (11) 20–23.

Chapter 8

Compassionate coaching in supervision: Residential care homes for older people

Andy Bradley

Introduction

Pain and suffering is a feature of our everyday lives and is felt as a direct result of our loss and our grief – there is an undercurrent of unexpressed grief in residential care and nursing homes as the care team may place emphasis on the physical and mental needs of the people they are caring for. The emotional and spiritual life of older people in care can be unexplored, leaving people feeling at a deeper level that they don't matter. Care teams are often stretched to the limit and so are preoccupied by the 'doing' aspects of care, as they lack space to enter the domain of 'being'. Slowing down, being still, listening, offering a comforting touch by holding a hand, a hand on a shoulder or even a hug are precious gifts which may be all too rarely available.

The experience of older people in care homes is frequently one of cumulative losses – of place, identity, control, valued relationships, community connection, confidence and in many cases, physical or mental capability. The paradigm in which care work takes place reinforces these losses; managers and care teams learn about safeguarding and manual handling as part of a tick box culture that leaves little room for reflecting on humanity, compassion, dignity and even love.

Fear may prevent residents and care workers opening up to each other as one may not trust the other to handle their feelings; emotions are often buried deeply as a consequence of adapting to an environment in which expressing feelings is not encouraged and validated. Residents may keep up a façade to their families in claiming they are content, because revealing the true extent of their pain may feel overwhelming.

To begin to create a new culture of listening, making space for older people to express what is in their hearts requires a radical shift of thinking – can we imagine a future in which care homes transform into thriving, humane, compassionate communities in which all belong, are known and safe?

As a manager in a care home to people with learning disabilities, and before that an NHS day centre, part of my role was to write the rota – despite my best efforts to recruit the right people for the job, to supervise the staff to enable them to grow and to lead the team to realise our vision, I was always more comfortable with the way some staff related to the people

we were caring for than others – there was a compassion gap in some. At that time I was using a conventional approach to supervision – for many of the people I managed this worked well, but I had a feeling that we were missing a deeper connection and purpose.

Morrison (2008) defines supervision as: *'a process in which one worker is given responsibility by the organisation to work with another worker(s) in order to meet certain organisational, professional and personal objectives.'* In this conventional supervision model the supervisor is tasked with keeping the supervisee on track – ensuring they are competent and accountable, that they feel well supported, are developing and that they are engaged with the organisation they work for. Compassionate coaching is based on the rationale that a sustainable compassionate and inclusive approach to care is not suited to what is effectively a performance management and employee engagement approach.

The evolution of compassion coaching

Having concluded that conventional approaches to supervision may not be suitable for all who work in residential care, reading, personal experience and reflection led to the development of the compassionate coaching approach. The extent to which the care worker is connecting with the person they are caring for is directly linked to their state of mind – the care worker could be absent or present as they offer care to another person. Jon Kabat-Zinn, a leading thinker globally on mindfulness whose work culminated in the development of the mindfulness based stress reduction programme, defines mindfulness as:

> *'The ability to pay attention to the present moment, on purpose without judgement.'* (Jon Kabat-Zinn, 1990)

Compassion coaching offers an opportunity to be in the moment with the person being coached, thereby modelling the kind of quality of attention that enables people to thrive – purposefully and without judgement. In this sense, compassion coaching is quite different from conventional supervision where the supervisor may come with a personal agenda which will inevitably, to some degree, influence how valuable and helpful the experience is for the supervisee. This is not to say that there is no place for conventional supervision, offering as it does a clear framework as described above. However, the conviction that lies behind the evolution of compassion coaching is that people who are caring for a living are likely to benefit from a different kind of space in which they have time to think and feel and an opportunity to reflect in the moment without fear of being judged.

The work of Professor Paul Gilbert of the Compassionate Mind Foundation is grounded in evolutionary psychology and that how our brains and behaviours have developed helps us to understand the challenges we face in being consistently compassionate to each other. We tend to default into a state of fear and emotional distance (triggered by the fight or flight stress response when we perceive ourselves to be unsafe or under threat) rather than into a more confident, consistent state of compassion. To be consistently compassionate at this stage in our evolution requires us to be conscious – we are tribal beings with a tendency for what Professor Gilbert calls 'kin preference', meaning we may back away from each other. The risk of this emotional distancing is heightened when one of us is caring for another, as our unspoken fears about our own vulnerability and mortality may be playing out and preventing us from offering our total compassionate presence.

Professor Gilbert's work described the three systems which are operating within us: the threat system, the doing system and the safety (or soothing) system. To be in a stable state of compassion these three systems need to be in balance. Care workers often report feelings of being overwhelmed by the pressure of caring tasks and anxious about 'getting it right' in an environment that may be driven more by the forces of competition and regulation than those of compassion and humanity. The intention to offer compassionate coaching is a conscious antidote to these forces, creating a safe caring space for honest personal reflection and opening up the potential for personal change and growth.

Health benefits for care workers

It is worth emphasising the health bringing benefits of caring with compassion – the narrative around emotional labour and care worker burn out suggests that caring over time can become overwhelming and unsustainable leading to a natural distancing response.

'Emotional labour is a serious problem faced by healthcare staff who strive to provide compassionate care. The ability to manage it is central to the provision of the best possible care while supporting staff well-being.' (Sawbridge & Hewison, 2014)

However the science suggests otherwise – it seems we are wired to be kind and that being in a compassionate state is good for us because as our vagal nerve fires, heart variability decreases and oxytocin (sometimes known as the 'yummy hormone' released through affection and breast feeding) is released.

'When you perform an act of kindness, especially when it involves face-to-face contact with the person involved, the momentary connection between you generates oxytocin in both you and them'. (Hamilton, 2010)

Being persistently threatened and overworked can mean overproducing adrenalin, cortisol and testosterone. A compassionate coach is aware of the need to downregulate the production of these hormones by being attentive to the needs of

the care worker, listening without judgement, being authentically curious about their experience and offering encouragement and appreciation for the care they give. Caring with compassion is intrinsically rewarding, and as has been said, good for our health, but the physical and emotional demands placed on care workers cannot be overstated – one-to-one compassion coaching is a valuable opportunity to validate and affirm the experience and commitment of care workers.

A structure for compassion coaching

Gilbert (2009) talks about the two psychologies of compassion and the way in which compassion flows. The first psychology is to be aware of suffering, the second is to be moved to act to alleviate the suffering in some way – being aware that another person is suffering may create an emotional response but it is only having the courage to act which means compassion is being expressed. Compassion has been defined as:

'Sensitivity to the distress of self and others with a commitment to try to do something about it and prevent it.' (Gilbert & Cole-King, 2012)

The activation of the two psychologies can lead to the flow of compassion in three ways:

→ Self to self.

→ Self to other.

→ Other to self.

Generally speaking, as a group, care workers tend to externalise their compassion, reserving what they have for 'self to other' compassion and find it more challenging to be compassionate to themselves or to accept compassion from others to them. Compassion that is only offered outwards may feel a little like pity as it is unequal and reserved only for those who are seen as more evidently needy. Compassionate coaching is challenging because the structure on offer creates space for reflection on the flow of compassion in all three domains.

Having developed a rationale for a more consciously compassionate approach to supervision, why integrate compassion with coaching rather than aligning compassion with supervision? Tim Gallwey, who has been very influential in developing the philosophy and practice of coaching in elite sports and other fields, says that the way for us to grow our competency and capacity is to reduce internal interference.

'People have more potential than they think they do – so the job of the coach is to reduce interference and grow potential.' (Gallwey, 2012)

The compassionate coach seeks to enable the coachee to understand the internal (and external) factors that may be preventing them from being part of the flow of compassion.

The qualities and behaviours of the compassionate coach

The compassionate coach offers a quality of attention and genuine care that they hope the care worker will in turn offer to residents, families and colleagues, and acknowledges the very real world challenges the care worker faces physically, mentally, emotionally and spiritually. '*I am here (present) - caring about you and your experience and believing you have the capacity to grow.*'

If you think of yourself as a skilful and patient gardener you will know that the compassion coaching structure is there to liberate, to help you to prepare the ground, till the soil, to sow seeds and make space for the people you are coaching to flourish and grow. Compassion coaching requires patience, trust and the positive assumption that given the right conditions we can all grow.

Compassionate coaching offers a space in which we can reflect on what struggles we face in being more human and look at what blocks our compassion and what releases it – starting with the compassion we feel for ourselves. The compassion coach begins by listening, making space for the coachee to mindfully consider the state they are in as they care. Three simple principles whose roots can be found in the practice of mindfulness guide the approach of the compassionate coach:

1. Listening with a quiet mind.

2. Asking questions that matter.

3. Appreciating from the heart.

It is crucial that the compassion coach has sufficient resources and is supported themselves, is part of the flow of compassion, is caring for themselves, is accepting compassion from others and ready to respond compassionately. Many of the people we meet who manage care homes have found thinking about the way they care for themselves confronting, uncomfortable and even at times distressing initially, but those who have gone on to become more active in self-care have described an increased capacity for offering a compassionate presence to the people they lead.

On a training seminar where the compassion coaching techniques were being modelled by the trainer with a nurse, a senior leader, when reflecting on the experience commented, '*Why hasn't everyone got access to that* [compassion coaching] *and why haven't I?*'

The leader went on to share that her supervision starts with a very brief question about her well-being before focusing primarily on firefighting, with complaints, grievances and safeguarding cases routinely taking up the bulk of her supervision time. There is no question that these are pressing and important managerial issues but the danger is that those who are tasked with being a leader in care services are left without a safe space to reflect and re-focus on how they will continue to care for themselves and others. Reactive management of this kind can lead to a toxic system in which the flow of compassion is systematically blocked.

The flow of compassion cannot be forced – it may be helpful for the compassion coach to see themselves as a gentle catalyst for change; building trust over time, discovering what enables the coachee to flourish and be happy and offering a consistent caring presence. The compassion coach knows that caring for people at the end of their lives asks a great deal of those who provide the care and that they are wise to be open to the vulnerability and pain that may be lying beneath the surface. Compassion coaches need to be humble and grounded, not seeking to advise or fix, and they are disciplined in ensuring they remain connected to the experiences of the people they are leading.

Outside of more formal one-to-one time for compassion coaching, the compassionate leader knows that they must get to know the people that care and the lives they lead outside of their caregiving role. Asking them why they do what they do, about their situation and their family and perhaps the story of compassion in their life signals a depth of care and a feeling that everyone in the community matters. This curiosity is the first step to building trust and creates the conditions in which deeper reflection on the growth of compassion becomes possible.

Finally, the compassion coach is full of courage (cour meaning heart). They are wholehearted in the way they lead, taking the risk of really getting to know the people doing the caring so that they can respond to the suffering they witness and build a culture based on a premise that everyone matters.

Structure of compassion coaching session

Recognising that care and nursing homes are often time-poor with pressure on carers to be continually available to care, for compassion coaching to be valuable it needs to be offered consistently as the benefits are found in frequency and gentle listening. Compassion coaching sessions work best when offered for a relatively short period of time such as 30 minutes, perhaps once a month.

The compassion coach should ensure that a quiet space conducive for thinking is available and should ensure the session will not be interrupted – glasses of water and a box of tissues should be routinely available.

After settling down, the coach may invite a moment or two of quiet to enable both parties to have a sense of arriving and being present before thanking the coachee for attending and saying a few words to set the scene.

To enter a positive frame of mind the coach can ask the coachee to share one thing that is going well outside of work – in the spirit of equality the coach should share something going well from their own perspective.

The process for the compassion coaching session then begins with space for reflection on self-compassion before moving on to thoughts regarding compassion for residents/service users and then the flow of compassion between team members.

The compassion coach begins with self-compassion and listens without interrupting while the coachee thinks and answers questions, for example:

→ What are your thoughts on how you have been caring for yourself?

→ What changes (if any) are you thinking of making to the way that you are caring for yourself?

→ What support or encouragement (if any) to make these changes would you like?

The coach should then move onto creating space for thoughts on compassion for residents:

→ What are your thoughts on how you have been caring for residents?

→ What changes (if any) are you thinking of making to the way that you are caring for residents?

→ What support or encouragement (if any) to make these changes would you like?

Finally the coach moves on to space for the coachee to think about the flow of compassion in the team:

→ What are your thoughts on how you and colleagues have been caring for each other?

→ What changes (if any) are you thinking of making to the way that you are caring for colleagues or what changes would you like to see in the way the team cares for each other?

→ What support or encouragement (if any) to make these changes would you like?

In each of the three domains of compassion the coach may deepen the enquiry by asking what might be preventing the flow of compassion or what might enable compassion to flow more readily. The compassion coach should make concise notes on the responses of the coachee, particularly around changes they say they would like to make and encouragement/ support requested.

The coach is listening for the growth of awareness and insight in the coachee; enabling them to find their own way of compassion. The coach may offer non-judgemental, encouraging reflections and specific appreciation (unless there are real concerns about the care workers approach) so that the care worker can hear how they are seen by the coach and can feel more confident and valued as a result.

The session ends with both parties having an opportunity to say what they have most appreciated about the session before agreeing a date for the next meeting. The coach ensures the coachee has a copy of notes of what has been agreed and future sessions include a recap and review.

The experience of offering compassion coaching in this way leads us to recommend that the coach holds the structure with time limited periods for thinking. This ensures that all three domains of compassion are considered and tends to leave the coachee feeling that they have enjoyed an opportunity to think through care and compassion in an integrated way and to find areas for intention around change.

Conclusion

Compassion coaching has the potential to help to break down barriers and to build relationships and alignment between professionals. In evolutionary terms we are tribal, and as a result we tend to negatively judge each other and focus on our differences in approaches and core values. This can make effective interprofessional team working a challenge. Compassion is all around us and within us – the challenge is to create the conditions in which compassion can flow, in which our better, kinder nature can be expressed. Moving beyond the dominant, linear, line manager performance management paradigm opens up possibilities for new, more reciprocal and nurturing relationships to flourish. A nurse could offer compassion coaching to a social worker and the social worker could offer the same space in return. Compassion is a uniting value and expressing our caring concern for each other by making the time and space to listen attentively without judgement would lead to more relational and integrated approach.

References

Gallwey T (2012) *Association for Coaching Interview* [online]. Available at: https://www.youtube.com/watch?v=q8X0v1NgXgQ (accessed November 2015).

Gilbert P (2009) *The Compassionate Mind*. London: Constable Publishing.

Gilbert P & Cole-King A (2012) Compassionate care: the theory and the reality. *Journal of Holistic Healthcare* **9** (3) 29–37.

Hamilton DR (2010) *Why Kindness is Good For You*. London: Hay House.

Kabat-Zinn J (1990) *Full Catastrophe Living – how to cope with stress, pain and illness using mindfulness meditation*. London: Piatkus Books.

Morrison (2008) *Supervision Policy, Standards and Criteria. Regional Policy for Northern Ireland, Health and Social Care Trusts* [online]. Department of Health, Social Services and Public Safety. Available at: http://www.dhsspsni.gov.uk/supervision_policy__standards__and_criteria___regional_policy_for_northern_ireland_health_and_social_care_trusts.pdf (accessed November 2015).

Sawbridge & Hewison (2014) Making Compassionate Care the Norm Starts with Our Staff. Online Commentary. *Health Service Journal*.

Chapter 9

Schwartz Rounds: What are they and how do they support all staff groups working in healthcare?

Rhiannon Barker and Dr Esther Flanagan

The need for support amongst healthcare staff

Healthcare staff are confronted with brutal situations on a regular basis. For instance patients and families angered by long waiting times or delayed discharge, patients suffering drawn out and sometimes painful deaths, increasingly complex clinical presentations and the daily pressures of working in under-resourced settings. These are just a few examples of the challenges faced by healthcare staff. It is therefore unsurprising that self-reported stress and sickness absence of health service staff is greater than that of the general population (Jones et al, 2013). Doctors have higher rates of mental health problems (depression, anxiety, alcohol or substance addictions and burnout) compared with the general population (Brooks et al, 2011) and 38% of nurses reported feeling unwell as a result of work-related stress in the past year (Royal College of Nursing, 2013). Yet, while forms of organisational support and supervision have been shown to bolster the drive for improved quality and safety of patient care, good examples of robust support are scant. Where good practice is identified it is often under threat of being squeezed out by regulatory and managerial demands (Tomlinson, 2015). In this chapter we will explore the value of Schwartz Rounds as an effective tool to foster and encourage staff support.

Staff experience has been shown to affect patient experience. Analysis of survey data from over 150,000 NHS staff and patients found that factors such as staff stress and additional working hours predicted poorer patient experience, whereas good managerial support for staff predicted improved patient experience (Raleigh et al, 2009). Dixon-Woods et al (2014) found that good staff support and management are linked to organisational culture and also relate to patient experience and quality of care. Goodrich and Cornwell (2008) outlined numerous individual and organisational elements of staff experience such as staff morale, support, accountability and health status, all of which can affect the quality of patient experience. This is supported by evidence that suggests positive staff experiences are linked to decreased absenteeism

(Powell et al, 2014), quality of care and patient satisfaction (Boorman, 2009). Interestingly, one study demonstrated that staff well-being (both physical and emotional health) was an antecedent to patient experience rather than a consequence, which further emphasises the need to pay attention to the well-being of healthcare staff (Maben et al, 2012). It seems logical to assume that in order for staff to deliver high quality care, they need to feel well in themselves, and one way of improving staff experience is to introduce greater support for them.

Historically, healthcare staff have supported one another over cups of tea during a lull in activity on the ward or in a chance corridor meeting. The term 'informal communities of coping' has been used to describe the means by which front-line service staff develop informal mechanisms in the form of 'collective emotional labour'. Korczynski (2003) describes the value of informal support networks of nurses and medical social workers, ascribed to the public venting of what are often deemed to be inappropriate emotions.

'Rest rooms, galleys, corridors and other "off-stage" areas provide an opportunity to employees to drop their corporate mask, free from the scrutiny of supervisors and customers. "Undesirable" emotions such as fear, anger, hurt and frustration can be vented or expressed… in the presence of a "willing" audience of colleagues.'
(Korczynski, 2003, p84)

These informal sources of support are valuable, but as demands build within 21st century healthcare environments, shared staff time is often pushed aside in the face of competing priorities. The design of big new modern hospitals may also impact on the ability of staff to work effectively together. A UK hospital was used as a case study for a two-year project that examined the impact of the interior design. They moved the setup from large bays and traditional 'Nightingale-style' wards to single room accommodation each with an ensuite bathroom (Maben et al, 2015). Staff reported that the single room accommodation made it harder for them to find other staff members and a reduction in contact with colleagues meant that it was more difficult to observe others' work, share ideas or ask for help.

The introduction of technology has increased the pace of organisational activities and could well have led to a reduction in face-to-face conversations and connections. While the pace and demands of 21st century healthcare have intensified, some cultural barriers to emotional expression and support in healthcare remain. In 1960, Isabel Menzies Lyth described how defences against distressing work were used by staff and enabled by organisations in the form of emotional withdrawal (e.g. working with symptoms not people) and the ability to hide behind professional roles and organisational targets.

> 'Often the patient's ill-being will evoke difficult feelings in the worker, sometimes in very obvious ways, like felt disapproval, overprotectiveness, anger or fear, and sometimes more obscurely, with subtler disturbances to engagement, empathy or response.' (Ballatt & Campling, 2011, p56)

These defences were reinforced by organisations as they were seen to protect staff against the emotional burden of care. The danger was that over time such defences created distance between staff and patients; when staff pulled away from seeing patients as individuals it was more difficult to deliver compassionate care. This suggests that compassion is, in part, enabled by seeing patients as people. Bilton and Cayton (2013) explored similar factors in relation to patient safety. They attempted to understand patient safety breaches using findings from Zimbardo's infamous Stanford prison experiment in 1973 (Haney et al, 1973). When a group of students were randomly assigned the role of 'guard' or 'prisoner' in a simulated prison, the 'guards' very quickly demonstrated an ability to inflict harm on the 'prisoners'. Zimbardo concluded that the behaviour demonstrated by the 'guards' was not due to flawed or immoral characters but the influence of the system in which they found themselves. He proposed that two conditions need to be in place for abusive behaviour to avail; 'deindividuation' of the perpetrators (a separation from personal identity), together with 'dehumanisation' of the maltreated.

> 'When identity is lost personal responsibility for one's actions is lost with it. In a professional setting, this is likely to result in a practitioner delivering unsafe care. In the light of these ideas we might want to draw parallels with care professionals not as the prison guards, but as themselves prisoners, subject to multiple, seemingly arbitrary and inconsistent orders, and thus becoming detached from decisions and judgements in which they should be fully engaged.' (Bilton and Cayton 2013, p9)

While Zimbardo's experiment focused on extreme behaviours, the findings resonate with some of the shocking abuses exposed in a number of hospital enquiries over the last decade (Francis, 2013). To protect against these conditions arising in healthcare environments, organisations should themselves treat staff with compassion and make sure adequate support mechanisms are in place.

The hierarchy of many work environments can be an additional barrier to effective working relations. Lachman (2013) suggests that entrenched, medicalised and hierarchical structures are a significant factor which discourage teamwork and transparency. The pressures

put on staff, working with people suffering increasingly complex co-morbidities, alongside the need to respond to emotional needs of patient and families, organisational demands and bureaucracies, can lead to adverse effects on clinicians' own well-being (Whitby et al, 2013).

Formal support for healthcare staff operates at a number of levels, normally within specific clinical disciplines. Psychologists, for example, undergo reflective practice and receive clinical supervision as a routine part of their job. Most professional forums in healthcare are made up of single professional groups such as psychologists or doctors. Multiprofessional clinical groups may also meet to look at clinical aspects of one particular case, but there are few forums where every staff member in an organisation is invited to attend, particularly non-clinical staff who also experience common stressors when working in healthcare settings. For example, receptionists are required to manage difficult and demanding patients; having to negotiate multiple roles as patient advocate, gatekeeper and even assessing the urgency of symptoms (Hammond et al, 2013; Eisner & Britten, 1999). But along with many other professionals, they are not routinely offered a forum to express the emotional impact of their work. Discussing the social and emotional aspects of care with colleagues across disciplines and positions, clinical and non-clinical, can help staff to understand shared challenges and foster a culture of connectedness. Schwartz Rounds, described below, are unique in offering reflective space to a broad, multiprofessional audience within health organisations.

What are Schwartz Rounds?

Schwartz Rounds provide a safe, confidential, voluntary, reflective forum for all staff, both clinical and non-clinical, to come together to discuss the emotional and social aspects of their jobs. The Rounds follow a standard model determining how they should be run, ensuring that they can be replicated across different settings. They normally take place once a month, for an hour at a time, usually at lunchtime with food provided. Food is an important sign that the staff are valued and cared for by the organisation. Audience numbers range from 20 to over 100 depending on the size of organisation. The basic format of the Rounds is that a panel of three or four staff members from different disciplines present stories of personal experiences. Their stories will relate to a particular topic, for example, 'giving bad news' or 'a patient I'll never forget'. Panellists take five minutes each to describe their story, focusing on how it made them feel and what emotional or social issues it raised for them. After the stories have been told and listened to, two trained facilitators open the discussion out to the audience. The facilitators guide the discussion, keeping it a reflective forum and drawing out themes from the audience's contributions. Schwartz Rounds are purely reflective, and the intention is that outcomes or solutions are not discussed. In healthcare, there is both individual and organisational pressure to identify solutions, so reflecting without solutions can feel new and perhaps uncomfortable.

Schwartz Rounds are not designed as a form of supervision and do not fit the traditional model of clinical supervision for several reasons: there is no expert and no advice is given, large groups of clinical and non-clinical staff attend, they do not focus on procedural or technical aspects of care, clinical outcomes or personal development. However, the Rounds do have some points of comparison with supervision: they may help to alleviate anxiety and normalise difficult emotions, they may impact on personal development indirectly through listening and sharing experiences with others and they help people to feel more supported in their role.

The history of Schwartz Rounds

In 1994 Kenneth Schwartz, a young health lawyer from Boston, was diagnosed with lung cancer. Before he died, he wrote a story about his care, in which he described the distress of the diagnosis and range of treatments he had to endure. But amongst the distress, Ken experienced moments of compassion and kindness from healthcare staff, which he highlighted as a vital part of care. He said:

'I have learned that medicine is not merely about performing tests or surgeries, or administering drugs…for as skilled and knowledgeable as my caregivers are, what matters most is that they have empathized with me in a way that gives me hope and makes me feel like a human being, not just an illness.' (Schwartz, 1995)

Kenneth did not want this human side to care to be neglected, so before his death, he left a legacy for the establishment of the Schwartz Center in Boston, to help to foster compassion in healthcare. This is where the Schwartz Rounds were developed and are currently running in over 300 organisations in the US. In 2009, Schwartz Rounds were brought to the UK by the Point of Care programme at The King's Fund and continue to be implemented by The Point of Care Foundation. In March 2014, over 115 healthcare organisations in the UK were signed up to run Rounds. Demand for Schwartz Rounds continues and has been driven in part by the favourable policy environment in the wake of the Darzi Review *High Quality Care for All: NHS next stage review* (Department of Health, 2008), The Mid Staffordshire NHS Foundation Trust Public Inquiry (Francis, 2013), which mentioned Schwartz Rounds as a means of supporting staff, the NHS England Business Plan (2014) that recommended them as an intervention to improve patient experience, and Delivering Dignity (Age UK, NHS Confederation & Local Government Association, 2012), which noted that staff must be given space to reflect on the care they deliver.

What is the evidence for Schwartz Rounds?

Evidence for Schwartz Rounds is growing alongside the number of organisations running them. There are two key studies that have quantitatively and qualitatively evaluated Rounds. Lown and Manning (2010) evaluated outcomes from US-based Schwartz Rounds using surveys and interviews. They looked at whether attending Rounds impacted on self-reported patient interaction and teamwork and found several changes, including increases in: a sense of compassion, energy, appreciation for other roles, connectedness to others, ability to manage sensitive and complex patient issues and insight into psychosocial elements of care. They also found a perceived decrease in stress and isolation. This study reported greater benefits in people who attended the Rounds regularly compared to those who did not. A UK study that analysed 41 interviews from acute hospital staff (Goodrich, 2012) supported the findings of the US study. Goodrich found that Rounds provided a space to validate concerns, mistakes and emotions

and also diminished hierarchies. Attendees felt that they were treated as equals and were able to observe senior staff talking openly about the emotional side of care. This helped to build a shared vision of support.

However, these two key studies are limited by self-reported outcome. A large scale, three year longitudinal study, which began in 2014, has been funded by the National Institute of Health Research. It attempts to identify mechanisms of Rounds and possible causal changes in a methodologically robust way that does not rely only on self-reported measures. It aims to uncover to what extent participation in Schwartz Rounds affects staff well-being, relationships between staff and patients and delivery of compassionate care. The study is entitled, *Supporting NHS staff at work: Could Schwartz Centre Rounds hold the key to a happier, healthier workforce and enhance compassionate care?* (National Institute for Health Research, 2014).

Rounds across healthcare settings

Schwartz Rounds began in relatively large sites providing acute care. But with the rapid expansion of Rounds they are now being introduced in a range of different clinical settings in the UK, including community and mental health trusts, hospices, primary care and educational settings. The Point of Care Foundation is exploring the logistical, operational and relational factors associated with these different settings, to examine which factors facilitate or impede progress. While there appears to be a number of generic factors influencing the success of the Rounds across all organisations, there are other, largely logistical issues, which may affect progress and uptake in more dispersed settings.

Where Rounds have got off to a good start the success is almost always linked to a committed and stable leadership team and early identification of a motivated, skilled, core Schwartz team who have been given permission, time and licence from the organisation to get the Rounds going. Having the capacity to demonstrate Rounds' benefits through shared stories and routine sharing of data is also key to continued support and momentum.

What are the mechanisms demonstrating how Schwartz Rounds work?

Attempts have been made to articulate the mechanisms responsible for the beneficial outcomes reported from the Rounds (Goodrich, 2012; Wren, 2014), yet a full theory remains undeveloped. Here we present six hypotheses covering various levels where their impact may be felt.

1. Normalising emotions

Healthcare settings can be lonely places, particularly if staff feel unsupported when coping with the difficult emotions that arise during the course of their work. Thoughts of fallibility, incompetence, bullying and feelings of fear, jealousy, grief and shame are all common experiences that are expressed during Schwartz Rounds. Sharing these experiences normalises them and allows staff to move from a place of isolation to a community of shared understanding. Normalisation in this context does not refer to diffusion or lessening emotion (as described in Ashforth & Humphrey, 1995), but rather in realising that unpleasant emotions are experienced by all, staff more openly express their own emotions. Normalising is recognised as a basic therapeutic skill in psychology, for validating others' experiences and reducing the sense of difference. When feelings are normalised, fears of personal failure and incompetence are reduced and there is a recognition that all people are prone to the same normal human fallibilities. This may help to overcome myths of healthcare staff as 'heroes' or 'automatons'. We suggest that in Rounds, the masks that help staff to defend against their daily work struggles are taken off and the person in the professional is revealed.

One nurse who attended a Round and heard a senior consultant talk of his/her own vulnerabilities reported:

'It's been so valuable hearing from different professional groups and learning that they too are vulnerable. When I was a newly qualified nurse there was one consultant who I was so terrified of. I used to hide in the toilets so that I wouldn't have to accompany them on the ward round. If I'd known at the time that consultants had the same emotions as me then I wouldn't have had to hide myself away!' (Nurse at Round)

2. Changing narratives

Stories have the ability to empower both narrator and audience. The power of telling and witnessing stories has been formalised in some psychological interventions. In Narrative Therapy (White & Epston, 1990), for example, the patient invites someone to witness their story and subsequently listens to the witness's response. This approach hypothesises that having an external observer helps us to validate our identity. Narratives move from being isolated and internal, to being shared and changeable. New narratives may also help staff to reconnect with their values; reaffirming the motivation behind working in the healthcare profession. As well as individual narratives, healthcare organisations as a whole will harbour narratives and therefore Rounds may help to populate the colour of the organisational narrative. For example, one story told by a porter in an acute trust rapidly spread across the organisation and changed the perception of a porter's role. The porter told of how he had been called to take a baby who had died to the mortuary and described the mother not wanting to let go of her child. The porter gently persuaded the mother to let the baby go by asking her to accompany him to the mortuary and reassuring her that he would take care of the baby. In the eyes of those attending the Round the role of the porter was transformed from a 'transporter' to someone who was integral to care and patient experience.

The Rounds may have the power to change narratives and in turn change the way people interact with one another.

'Everything just slightly tilts, and the next time you see them you're different with them from how you were before, and if what they are saying resonates with you, you feel you have a different connection with them.' (Nurse at a Round, from Reed et al, 2014)

3. Promoting connectedness

Healthcare environments are increasingly fragmented, hierarchical and tribal places, with each professional carrying out their own duties, but not necessarily with a sense of how their contribution connects with the complete patient journey. The Rounds appear to engender a sense of connectedness with the 'whole' system.

'I sometimes feel as if you're a little part of a jigsaw and going to a Schwartz Round you see all the other bits of the jigsaw, so you actually get the whole picture which is ... it's reassuring, it's comforting, it's enlightening, it's educational, it's all these things.' (Volunteer at Round, from Reed et al, 2014)

Currently, Schwartz Rounds are the only forum that allow healthcare staff at all levels and from all departments to come together in a reflective space. Having a diverse mix of staff groups engaging in dialogue allows for a deeper understanding of each others' roles and a stronger sense of connectedness. In turn, the hierarchies that are often strongly pronounced within medicine are temporarily, or possibly more permanently, flattened (Goodrich, 2012). This links back to the 'person in the professional'; once the person is revealed, staff may connect more easily as human beings.

One social worker who attended a Round said:

'You don't feel quite so alone. I think sometimes when we're very stretched you feel it's just you, you know, it's just you that's carrying this burden and then you realise that actually the whole team is around you and they're carrying it too.' (Social worker at Round, The Point of Care Foundation, 2014)

4. Creating a culture of openness

Schwartz Rounds not only create connections between individuals, but may contribute to a wider culture of openness. The discussions that occur in Rounds model new modes of interaction, in which staff can share experiences without judgement or solutions.

'I've been interested listening to the various contributions how many of my own emotions it's unlocked. Emotions that were deeply buried within me. I think we all tend to do this and the danger of locking things away is that you then don't recognise these feelings when other people are going through them.' (Consultant at hospital Round, The Point of Care Foundation, 2014)

Over time, this consistent reflective space may impact on the organisation more broadly, encouraging staff to employ their reflective stance in their work outside the Round. For example, staff often disclose experiences of fallibility and mistakes in Rounds; if this is carried across into their everyday practice or work, a culture of increased openness and transparency could develop.

5. The 'failure to cure'

Healthcare services and staff are often judged on their ability to 'cure'. Improving health is the fundamental purpose of healthcare, however sometimes patients cannot be healed. This not only applies to end of life care, but to populations with chronic physical and mental health conditions, in which improvement is sometimes difficult to achieve. Gawande (2014) in his book *Being Mortal* describes the tendency of the medical profession to want to fight death at all costs, often without honest consideration of what this means to the patient's deteriorating quality of life. Yet, he reminds us, death eventually wins. He advises:

'You don't want a general who fights to the point of total annihilation. You don't want Custer. You want

Robert E. Lee, someone who knows how to fight for territory that can be won and how to surrender it when it can't, someone who understands that the damage is greatest if all you do is battle to the bitter end.' (Gawande, 2014, p187)

Gawande highlights with great sensitivity the difficulties that healthcare staff have in facing issues of immortality and of initiating the discussions that need to be had with patients to help them make decisions around their treatment and care. Schwartz Rounds are a rare opportunity to tackle some of the unresolved issues that healthcare staff feel, e.g. when patients can't be 'cured' or have been treated by a series of brutal and possibly ineffective interventions. The Rounds can provide a space for staff to reconnect with the importance of open communication and demonstrate that kindness and empathy (not just clinical outcomes) are integral to good quality care.

6. Role modelling

More than a century ago William Osler proposed a model of medical education based largely on teaching by example (Scott *et al*, 1998). Today, role modelling continues to be seen as integral both to medical education and the ongoing acquisition of professional skills. Schwartz Rounds can provide opportunities for positive role modelling and the promotion, through example, of good professional practice; specifically related to the more human side of care. Junior staff and students may in particular find it useful to witness senior staff reflect on the emotional side of care, which is often masked by professional barriers and entrenched hierarchies.

'…that surgeon is so high up I would normally be intimidated by him. I'm a medical student and don't want to say anything stupid, but his presentation made him so much more approachable. So if I now had him [for a teacher] and you find a situation upsetting you would be much more likely to say something or be more open with him. Not to be so scared to say something … it's good bridging.' (Medical student attending a Round)

Rounds won't work for everyone

We have looked at mechanisms that may work to accrue positive benefits of attending Rounds. But it is important to acknowledge that Rounds won't suit everyone and people have different styles of coping with the emotional burden of care.

'Some people cope by pushing things to the side – that's OK – it's one way of coping. There is no right or wrong way. We don't need to judge. In order to build your own resilience everyone needs to find their own way.' (Round facilitator)

Conclusion

This chapter has highlighted the need for more formalised forms of emotional support for staff working in health care settings and has showcased Schwartz Rounds as an evidence-based way of helping to alleviate some of the stress, anxiety and sense of fragmentation that can build up. The unique potential of Schwartz Rounds to offer support for all groups of staff in a non-hierarchical forum has been particularly appreciated by those involved. The experience is levelling and offers a rare insight into the emotional impact of the everyday routine on healthcare staff. Porters, secretaries, consultants, nurses, allied health professionals, catering staff, all come together and offer a glimpse of the stresses and strains of each other's lives. The recognition of different roles within the organisations and the ability to see the person in the profession helps build team cohesion. The conversations that unravel appear to impact at an individual, team and organisational level, highlighting that all staff contributions are integral to the overall ambition of improved patient outcomes.

While Rounds can't be equated to supervision, they share a number of common outcomes, specifically relating to an increased sense of support, alleviating anxieties and normalising emotions. The clearly defined model for running Rounds is welcomed by users and ensures replicability across settings. The outcomes from Rounds are generally perceived positively by staff, though the complexities of the different contexts in which they are operationalised present challenges and there are notable factors that may hinder successful implementation. Importantly, Rounds require top level support; organisations need to prioritise resources to set them up and sustain them and to encourage and enable attendance by everyone.

Their rapid growth in the UK is to be celebrated and is a clear demonstration of the need for improved staff support. While the Rounds were first developed within acute trusts, they are now running in a variety of settings including: hospices community trusts, mental health trusts, an ambulance trust and a medical school. There is growing interest shown in the model from a number of different sectors including education and business. We are in the process of building a more coherent framework, articulating the mechanisms at work during the Rounds and demonstrating how successful outcomes can be routinely achieved across a variety of different settings. One of our particular ambitions is to develop a cost-effective model which can be implemented in organisations where opportunities for support and reflection are at best limited, and where staff numbers are comparatively small, such as GP practices. It is hoped that the growing body of data and evidence being collected, coupled with the National Institute for Health Research study currently underway, will contribute to an even more robust evidence base.

References

Age UK, NHS Confederation and Local Government Association (2012). *Delivering Dignity* [online]. Available at: http://www.ageuk.org.uk/Global/Delivering%20Dignity%20Report.pdf?dtrk=true (accessed November 2015).

Ashforth BE & Humphrey RH (1995) Emotion in the workplace: a reappraisal. *Human Relations* **48** (2) 97–125.

Ballatt J & Campling P (2011) *Intelligent Kindness: Reforming the culture of healthcare*. London: RCPsych Publications.

Bilton D & Cayton H (2013) *Asymmetry of Influence: The role of regulators in patient safety* [online]. London: The Health Foundation. Available at: http://www.health.org.uk/sites/default/files/AysmmetryOfInfluenceTheRoleOfRegulatorsInPatientSafety.pdf (accessed November 2015).

Boorman (2009) *NHS Health and Well-being Review* [online]. Department of Health. Available at: http://webarchive.nationalarchives.gov.uk/20130107105354/http://www.dh.gov.uk/en/

Publicationsandstatistics/Publications/PublicationsPolicyAndGuidance/ DH_108799 (accessed November 2015).

Brooks SK, Chalder T & Gerada C (2011) Doctors vulnerable to psychological distress and addictions: treatment from the Practitioner Health Programme. *Journal of Mental Health* **20** (2) 157–164.

Department of Health (2008) *NHS Next Stage Review* [online]. Available at: http://webarchive.nationalarchives.gov.uk/20130107105354/http:/ www.dh.gov.uk/prod_consum_dh/groups/dh_digitalassets/@dh/@en/ documents/digitalasset/dh_085826.pdf (accessed November 2015).

Dixon-Woods M, Baker R, Charles, K, Dawson J, Jerzembek G, Martin G, McCarthy I, McKee L, Minion J, Ozieranski P, Willars J, Wilkie P & West M (2014) Culture and behaviour in the English National Health Service: overview of lessons from a large multimethod study. *BMJ Quality & Safety* **23** (2) 106–115.

Eisner M & Britten N (1999) What do general practice receptionists think and feel about their work? *British Journal of General Practice* **49** (439) 103–106.

Francis R (2013) *Report of the Mid Staffordshire NHS Foundation Trust Public Inquiry: Executive summary* (Vol. 947). London: The Stationery Office. Available at: https://www.gov.uk/government/uploads/system/ uploads/attachment_data/file/279124/0947.pdf (accessed November 2015).

Gawande A (2014) *Being Mortal*. Toronto: Doubleday Canada.

Goodrich J (2012) Supporting hospital staff to provide compassionate care: do Schwartz Center Rounds work in English hospitals? *Journal of the Royal Society of Medicine* **105** (3) 117–122.

Goodrich J & Cornwell J (2008) *Seeing the Person in the Patient*. London: The King's Fund.

Hammond J, Gravenhorst K, Funnell E, Beatty S, Hibbert D, Lamb, J, Burroughs H, Kovandžić M, Gabbay M, Dowrick C, Gask L, Waheed W & Chew-Graham CA (2013) Slaying the dragon myth: an ethnographic study of receptionists in UK general practice. *British Journal of General Practice* **63** (608) e177–e184.

Haney C, Banks WC & Zimbardo PG (1973) A study of prisoners and guards in a simulated prison. *Naval Research Review* **30** 4–17.

Jones MC, Wells M, Gao C, Cassidy B & Davie J (2013) Work stress and well-being in oncology settings: a multidisciplinary study of health care professionals. *Psycho-Oncology* **22** (1) 46–53.

Korczynski M (2003) Communities of coping: collective emotional labour in service work. *Organization* **10** (1) 55–79.

Lachman P (2013) Redefining the clinical gaze. *BMJ Quality & Safety* **22** (11) 888–890.

Lown BA & Manning CF (2010) The Schwartz Center Rounds: evaluation of an interdisciplinary approach to enhancing patient-centered communication, teamwork, and provider support. *Academic Medicine* **85** (6) 1073–1081.

Maben J, Griffiths P, Penfold C, Simon M, Pizzo E, Anderson J, Robert G, Hughes J, Murrells T, Brearley S & Barlow J (2015) Evaluating a major innovation in hospital design: workforce implications and impact on patient and staff experiences of all single room hospital accommodation. *Health Services and Delivery Research* **3** (3).

Maben J, Peccei R, Adams M, Robert G, Richardson A, Murrells T & Morrow E (2012) *Exploring the Relationship Between Patients' Experiences of Care and the Influence of Staff Motivation, Affect and Wellbeing* [online]. Final report. UK National Institute for Health Research Service Delivery and Organisation Programme. Available at: http://www.netscc.ac.uk/hsdr/files/project/SDO_FR_08-1819-213_V01. pdf (accessed November 2015).

Menzies Lyth I (1960) Social systems as a defense against anxiety: an empirical study of the nursing service of a general hospital. *Human Relations* **13** (2) 95–121.

National Institute for Health Research (2014) *Protocol: A Longitudinal National Evaluation of Schwartz Centre Rounds: An intervention to enhance compassion in relationships between staff and patients through providing support for staff and promoting their well-being* [online]. Available at: http://www.nets.nihr.ac.uk/__data/assets/ pdf_file/0004/129631/PRO-13-07-49.pdf (accessed November 2015).

NHS England (2014) *Putting Patients First: The NHS England business plan for 2014/15 – 2016/17* [online]. The NHS Constitution. Available at: http://www.england.nhs.uk/wp-content/uploads/2014/04/ppf-1415-1617-wa.pdf (accessed November 2015).

Powell M, Dawson J, Topakas A, Durose J & Fewtrell C (2014) Staff satisfaction and organisational performance: evidence from a longitudinal secondary analysis of the NHS staff survey and outcome data. *Health Services and Delivery Research* **2** (50).

Raleigh VS, Hussey D, Seccombe I & Qi R (2009) Do associations between staff and inpatient feedback have the potential for improving patient experience? An analysis of surveys in NHS acute trusts in England. *Quality and Safety in Health Care* **18** (5) 347–354.

Reed E, Cullen A, Gannon C, Knight A & Todd J (2014) Use of Schwartz Centre Rounds in a UK hospice: findings from a longitudinal evaluation. *Journal of Interprofessional Care* **29** (4) 365–366.

Royal College of Nursing (2013) *Beyond Breaking Point: A survey report of RCN members on health, well-being and stress* [online]. Available at: http://www.rcn.org.uk/__data/assets/pdf_file/0005/541778/004448.pdf (accessed November 2015).

Schwartz KB (1995) A patient's story. *The Boston Globe Magazine* July 16. Available at: http://www.theschwartzcenter.org/media/patient_story. pdf (accessed November 2015).

Scott M, Wright MD, Kern DE, Kolodner K, Howard DM & Brancati FL (1998) Attributes of excellent attending-physician role models. *New England Journal of Medicine* **339** (27) 1986–1993.

The Point of Care Foundation (2014) *Staff Care: How to engage staff in the NHS and why it matters* [online]. Available at: http://www. pointofcarefoundation.org.uk/Downloads/Staff-Report-2014.pdf (accessed November 2015).

Tomlinson J (2015) Using clinical supervision to improve the quality and safety of patient care: a response to Berwick and Francis. *BMC Medical Education* **15** (103).

White M & Epston D (1990) *Narrative Means to Therapeutic Ends*. New York: WW Norton & Company.

Wren B (2014) Schwartz Rounds: an intervention with potential to simultaneously improve staff experience and organisational culture. *Clinical Psychology Forum* **263** 22–25.

Part III:

Despatches from the front-line: Service user and front-line practitioners' perspectives

Introduction to Part III

Part III presents some personal reflections on staff supervision from the perspectives of managers and service users. Two managers from social work and nursing respectively report on the realities at the front-line of trying deliver national and local policies in practice, and what it means to supervise staff from different professional backgrounds. While the final chapter deconstructs supervision as a hierarchal practice from the perspective of a service user researcher and disability rights activist.

In Chapter 10, Jeremy Winter, a register social worker and advanced practitioner, describes his experiences of managing an integrated team for adults with learning disability. Jeremy writes with great warmth about working with colleagues from a variety of backgrounds including community nurses, physiotherapists, psychology, speech therapy and behavioural support as well social workers. He describes a collaborative culture that fostered joint working between health and social care colleagues, cemented via interprofessional supervision as a means to share learning across disciplines. Jeremy firmly believes that this made a difference to outcomes for people using services.

Kevin Brett, registered nurse and manager, presents a somewhat contrasting set of experiences in Chapter 11. Kevin describes with verve the challenges of managing a team of social workers and nurses set up to deliver integrated care to older people with complex needs, yet struggling to provide the joined up approach envisaged in the face of confusing and contradictory systems. Interprofessional supervision was one means of building understanding between disciplines but needs to happen in a wider context where joint working is genuinely facilitated throughout the organisation.

In Chapter 12, Maryam Zonouzi, a service user researcher and award-winning social entrepreneur, challenges us to move beyond a hierarchal model of supervision that is about professionals 'watching over' practice, to a relational approach that is about 'watching between' service users, personal assistants and professionals. This chapter encourages us to break free from unhelpful binaries that define us as 'professional' or 'service user', 'employer' or 'employee' and focus on how we can build relationships and work better together to improve the lives of people using services.

Finally, Lisa Bostock reflects on the core themes of the book in Chapter 13, exploring the place of interprofessional supervision within the context of changing demographics, confusing service systems and constrained resources, before offering some suggestions about 'where next' for research on supervision in adult services.

Chapter 10

Interprofessional supervision: Building an environment of learning and trust in an integrated setting for people with learning disabilities

Jeremy Winter

For a period of almost two years from early 2007 until late 2008, I had the good fortune to be appointed to the role of assistant integrated manager of an adult integrated learning disability team in Lancashire. I say 'good fortune' because, having worked in a variety of arrangements of health and social care learning disability teams before that time and since, across all three local authorities in the broader Lancashire area, I am of the very definite opinion that this arrangement works best.

One of the reasons for this was the multidisciplinary nature of the team's management (the manager was employed by health and I was employed by social services), which led to the establishment of interprofessional supervision (IPS) arrangements for the staff, who came from a variety of professional disciplines – social workers, community nurses, speech therapists, physiotherapists, a clinical psychologist and a behavioural support team.

There were many reasons why, in my opinion, the team worked so well. The relationship between the integrated manager and myself was exceptionally good, which gave a certain stability to all the team members. We were very different personalities, but were able to appreciate each other's strengths and cover each other's weaknesses in a highly complementary way.

Prior to my appointment, I had worked on the team as an agency social worker for about six months, so I'd had the chance to get to know the workings of the team at close quarters. Previous to this I had also worked in two other multidisciplinary teams, so had gained some valuable experience of other disciplines' ways of working and their agenda, and had also had a manager employed by health for a number of years. I was perhaps ideally prepared, at this point in my career, to carry out the role to which I was appointed.

The team was, I believe, well organised and I arrived at a time when some poor practice had been rectified. Nevertheless, high workloads and an ever-changing health and social care agenda meant that we needed to work in an effective and efficient way, seeking to manage the increasing expectations of both the general public and our respective employers. IPS was already well established, meaning that new staff almost took it for granted, whereas I understand that in the early stages of the team this was not the case, with some professionals struggling to accept supervision from someone not from their discipline. This resistance was only gradually overcome by putting in a great deal of time and effort, carrying out our own independent research into the role and practice of those from a different professional background and training, and demonstrating a growing understanding of both health and social care work.

A weekly joint allocation meeting was already well-established as a high priority and the majority of the team usually attended. The task of chairing this lively session usually fell to me, with the aim of allocating all work to the relevant professional or professionals, in a timely manner. This meeting was the heart of the team in many ways, where a mixture of good humoured banter and managing incoming work enabled the team to function in a usually good natured way, allowing for different opinions to be voiced in an atmosphere of mutual respect.

The manager and I divided up most of the team with the exception of the speech and language therapist and the clinical psychologist, whom we consulted with, but were professionally not able to provide supervision to. This ensured that everyone received supervision on a regular basis. We decided that the team would work most effectively if we did not divide this task along professional lines, so each of us agreed to provide supervision to some health staff and some social care staff.

This would give both of us a close view of the work being undertaken by each discipline. Also, as the team developed, it gradually began to be accepted that staff would record on the same IT system and would carry out some of the same tasks (such as care management tasks, including some commissioning). This was not without its difficulties, for example, to allow nursing staff to record on the social services data base, while still satisfying the demands of their own profession, each entry had to be entitled 'nursing record'. Our negotiating skills, both with the staff and their respective management hierarchy, were, at times, stretched.

If I was providing supervision to a nurse, there were elements of their work that I was not very knowledgeable about. However I did not feel this detracted from the quality of the supervision, as long as I remained humble enough to be able to learn from them at these times. If there were health-related issues they needed guidance with, it was always possible to ask my manager for assistance; she also sought my assistance with social care issues on occasion. Both of us sought to learn as much as we could about the other discipline, so that the professionals developed some faith in our ability to provide them with competent, professional supervision.

Health staff also had to provide specific information to meet health-related performance indicators and this work had to be checked by the health manager. At that time, social workers had to have regard for performance indicators, but these were related to specific outcomes, rather than to their practice. However, since the advent of the Health and Care Professions Council as a regulatory body and the Performance Capability Framework, social workers also have to provide evidence of their competence. In today's health and social care arena, I think it would be necessary for there to be some input from relevant health and social care managers to support IPS.

IPS was perhaps at its best when a nurse and a social worker were jointly working a case, which happened often. Joint supervision, based around specific cases and involving both workers and one manager, either from health or social care, provided an effective and efficient way of providing professional direction. Being able to refer back to the manager from the other discipline on a regular basis provided some form of accountability to the staff. The mutual respect that existed between the two managers meant that decisions were respected and were only overturned for good reason and only rarely because of managerial hierarchy.

I believe this led to achieving better and often quicker outcomes for service users, though it is difficult to substantiate this. All I can point to are situations where poor joint working has frequently delayed outcomes being agreed. To me it stands to reason that if relationships between professionals of different disciplines are respectful, open and honest (which is more likely when this is being modelled by those in management positions), that the people we are there to serve will benefit in all kinds of ways, and are more likely to feel secure being cared for by a system which must appear bewilderingly complex at times. I also believe that IPS helped to achieve better working relationships between front-line professionals, improving communication and understanding of each other's roles.

Overall, IPSs were as challenging as they were enlightening and informative for both supervisor and practitioner, whatever the discipline. The challenges were not easy to manage on occasion, but they did not detract from the overall ethos of supervision and mutual respect. Over time in our multidisciplinary team, opinions, pathways, judgements and outcomes became more in line with each other the longer we worked together. This in turn produced closer working relationships where supervisions became more democratic and two-way, rather than autocratic or manager-led. Exceptions were where legislation needed to be adhered to and the practitioner needed guidance, although this was usually due to inexperience rather than incompetence.

I left to manage a social care adult learning disability team, co-located with a health team. I had hopes that these teams would eventually be integrated and I would be able to put my experience of the past couple of years to good use. However, despite some level of willingness to engage with this process at my level, relationships between strategic managers of both organisations in this area were somewhat strained, making integration unlikely.

Front-line staff had established some good working relationships, but health and social care staff sat in blocks separately to each other and there was, at times, interprofessional rivalry and envy. Looking back, I think this geographical area was busier than in my previous position, with more complex cases but without additional resources, and the team was recovering from long term managerial sickness. Even so, I don't believe either team ran as well as the integrated one had, to the detriment of staff and service users.

A further restructure in the local authority effectively broke up both the integrated team and the social care team to which I had moved, as generic working (with all adult service user groups caseloads) became the order of the day. I know that some staff from the old learning disability teams still hanker after returning to their specialism and I have spoken to several staff from the integrated team who think, as I do, that working in that way was one of the highlights of their career. In fact, since the time of writing we are about to revert to specialist learning disability teams again in Lancashire, from October 2015 – an announcement greeted with enthusiasm.

In 2014, I had occasion to attend a multidisciplinary county council meeting looking at learning disability services and there was some appetite there to work towards integration once more, despite the current prevailing view. Now, in 2015, the Care Act (2014) applies to both health and social care agencies and there is much talk in the current political debate about integrating the two, with Greater Manchester recently being given the go-ahead to do so. I have no doubt that other local authorities and clinical commissioning groups will be watching the progress of this with great interest. Even if this may be more motivated by having to manage increasing demands with fewer resources, I for one, from the experiences described, can see many advantages of working in this way. If it goes ahead, which looks promising, IPS is likely to become more common once again. I would argue that this is crucial to the success of overall integration, as each profession learns to trust the judgement and bow to the wisdom of the other. To quote my manager at the time, *'Interprofessional supervision is healthy; it fosters mutual professional respect, increases skills and knowledge and should be promoted within health and social care as gold standard practice.'*

Chapter 11

Supervision across interprofessional boundaries: A practitioner's perspective

Kevin Brett

I was appointed as an integrated service manager for a team of therapists, social workers and nurses based in the community, who are commissioned to reduce avoidable hospital admissions and facilitate safe and timely discharges across several acute trusts in the West Midlands. The aim of the team was to provide a more joined-up approach to meeting the complex needs of many of the elderly population we support in our locality. The team was unique within the trust as it was the first to provide a more seamless approach to health and social care by integrated working across professional boundaries, with shared goals and outcomes.

I joined the team approximately 18 months after it was commissioned, and was relishing the challenge of managing a group of people who were leading the way in meeting the government's strategy of a more effective system of managing the complex needs of an aging population to maintain their health and well-being in a variety of settings. I have a background in nursing, have worked as a ward manager for many years and understood the role and responsibilities of therapists and nurses, but social workers are an unknown quantity to me. I never had much contact with them unless it was part of a multidisciplinary team meeting or trying to decipher their notes in the medical records. The only training I have received in social care was listening to *Clare in the Community* on Radio Four. But I felt reassured my lack of knowledge and experience managing social workers would not be a hindrance as the team, I was reliably informed, manage themselves.

After a few days at work it was quickly apparent I was naive in believing I would be in charge of people from a variety of professional backgrounds who were all working together, putting aside professional and personnel differences, to meet the needs of individuals as a unified team. Some boxes were ticked in the trust's integration agenda, everyone was co-located in one building, there were shared facilities and people met once a month for a team meeting but that was more or less the extent of 'integration'. The portrayal of close working between health and social care did not match the reality; expecting a Walton's approach to sharing responsibilities and solving differences through dialogue and mutual respect, the reality was more like the Simpsons.

The team are hardworking, dedicated, are meeting the daily demands for their services with commitment, compassion and a high degree of professionalism, but watching them work 'together' was more like watching a busy child's playground, in the sense there was a lot of noise and activity but everyone was playing in parallel, no group activities, mixing with their own circle of friends with a few lone stragglers on the peripheries. This resulted in service users receiving conflicting advice regarding the type of care package they would be getting when there was a requirement for enablement following an assessment. The social worker might say they need physiotherapy, the physiotherapist may disagree or reduce their input and the occupational therapist would not conform to any care planning until the service user was assessed by them. However some individuals would agree to follow care plans and be guided by the initial assessments of the social worker, so the approach each profession took depended on who you talked to. A frequent complaint from service users was the care and support on offer did not match what was received.

The team's methodology and ways of working mirrored the trust's infrastructure across the whole organisation. Everyone swimming against a tide of complex and differing systems and processes that are not joined up and are full of jargon and terminology, making any shared documentation difficult to understand and hard to follow. Contacts were not aligned, therefore even managing leave and sickness, a staple requirement of any manager, required knowledge of separate policies depending on whether the person was under health or social terms and conditions. Changes are being made to pull everything together but it is slow; until recently I had two different email accounts and could not access my team leader's calendar, nor could they access mine.

To reinforce the lines of demarcation at a local level the notice boards in the building were marked 'health' and 'social', and even birthday collections were kept separate. While there will always be personal differences in any team, the natural separation into professional groups could be explained by the fact that culture and focus for social workers is different to that of health/therapy colleagues, lending itself for people to gravitate within their own professional boundaries. The principle of integration is sound and in many industries works well, but for health and social care it is the same as having apples and pears in the same bowl and calling them oranges. They will always taste, feel and look different despite how you try and change the labelling, though having them together does allow ease of access.

My focus to start bringing the team working closer together was to develop a model of co-operation and collaboration rather than integration, making it clear that changes were going to be made and things were going to be different. Low morale was also prevalent as many felt the work they were doing was not valued or understood, both within the team and by the organisations and professionals who made referrals to them. Unrealistic expectations regarding outcomes and timeframes from the referrers, and the resulting negative feedback when expectations were not met caused frustration and a feeling of helplessness.

A concentrated approach was made to focus on what we could change ourselves. Each individual in the team would provide mutual support for each other, developing a siege mentality with our base referred to as 'The Alamo', with us all joining together to become a strong and cohesive unit. I had a vision of an Olympic ring model of care where there is an overlap, with certain tasks carried out by anyone with the right skills and expertise. The starting point was to engage with the team and ask them what immediate changes they would like to make, this resulted in notice boards renamed 'team' and 'activities'. Birthdays were reorganised so everyone was included and on the activity board outings, events, special celebrations and achievements were promoted. As the workforce consisted of 80% women, toilet names were changed from 'male' and 'female' to 'staff', which was universally well received. The aim of this exercise was to create conversation between everyone where a consensus of opinion was reached, demonstrating we can all put aside professional rivalry to work together and benefit from the resulting outcomes.

The long term aim was to produce a multiprofessional team who were responsive, effective and worked well together. This required a bottom-up approach with top-down support allowing me a high degree of autonomy to make managerial decisions without going through a lengthy bureaucratic process. I see my role as both manager and leader; these are distinct yet interlinked in developing cross-boundary working, team cohesion and a shared vision and sense of purpose.

The managerial side of my role included ensuring that there were learning and development opportunities to help everyone understand each other's roles and responsibilities. This helped reduce misconceptions around who could do what, when many tasks were profession-specific and underpinned by clear lines of accountability. Each referral pathway was examined and mapped to find out areas where there could be a chance to work in the shaded areas of those Olympic rings. These exercises created debate, disagreement, but above all communication. The fundamental managerial principle instilled was that we all work in a no-blame culture, safety is paramount, but the team were allowed to start making their own solutions to managing demand with limited resources. Taking ownership in finding solutions makes sense as the team are the ones working on the coalface and therefore know what is needed to improve care and positive outcomes.

The leadership side of my role was to promote what we can do, not what we can't, and to help create an environment where everyone counts and there is always time to talk, listen and to develop an appreciative atmosphere. With any disputes or disagreements there was an expectation to either resolve the issue or agree to disagree, but still get on with the day job and not lose sight of the bigger picture; that we all needed to work together for the benefit of the service users. This would take precedence over personal or professional differences.

Supervision across professional boundaries is a challenge, especially when you do not have the background or training in the work half your workforce undertakes, but it can be achieved. It does help to have supporting policies to guide you through the process and ensure a degree of standardisation so that everyone knows what to expect from themselves and their supervisor, but above all understand the value of supervision and why it is important to the individual and the team. The trust also made it mandatory for supervision to be carried out, which was the stick, if needed, for anyone not willing to undertake or delay their supervision.

A key approach I use is promoting the benefits of having protected time to discuss and share concerns and areas of development and praise, which leads to positive outcomes and feelings of being supported and valued. This can be achieved across professional boundaries as dialogue is two-way and learning can be shared when it comes to profession-specific issues. I believe true integration is a concept rather than a reality; social work and nursing and therapy are distinctly different. However they do have a lot of commonality around providing help and support in meeting the holistic needs of individuals, and some aspects of professional roles can be developed. Interprofessional supervision is a key element in supporting effective, integrated team working. It provides the opportunity to build relationships and greater understanding between supervisor and supervisee in a safe environment, if done effectively and not seen by both parties as just something else to do.

Supervision for me has proved invaluable to gain feedback and guidance in how I approach my role as manager. Supporting the individual to reach their potential can only benefit the whole team and help it to reach its potential to provide safe, effective and high quality care, as any team is the sum of its individual parts.

Chapter 12

Service users and the supervision of personal assistants

Maryam Zonouzi

Since the Community Care (Direct Payments) Act (1996) there have been increased calls for social care to be responsive to the individual needs of service users. Direct payments mean local councils can now give cash directly to service users to make their own care arrangements, rather than the council arranging the service. Demand for greater choice and control led to the 'personalisation' agenda encompassing the idea of self-directed support in social care and self-management in healthcare. Successive social policies supported many service users to realise their aspiration for independent living (Evans, 2003), and supported the government's agenda to make citizens responsible for their own health and social care needs.

These policy shifts have changed the relationship between social care professionals (social workers), care and support workers and personal assistants (paid support) and service users. Professionals are now encouraged to support service users to procure their own care and to take management responsibility for care and support workers, previously the responsibility of local authorities whose purview is now the overall quality of procured services. As oversight, quality, pay, conditions and supervision have shifted away from professionals and local authorities to service users, little research has examined the impact of these shifts.

This chapter draws on 18 years' personal experience of managing my own direct payments and five years PhD research exploring the impact of shifts in responsibility from professionals to service users. Both my personal and academic endeavours underpin the rationale for reconceptualising supervision away from a hierarchical 'watching over' model towards intervision or 'watching between', representing a practical shift towards a relational approach between service users, personal assistants (PAs) and professionals. In this model, all participants jointly share accountability, status and responsibility.

The tangible steps laid out here have needed to take place politically and interpersonally to support a transition away from the hierarchical to relational intervision. Presenting the chapter in this way allows the reader to chart where they are on this journey and to critically examine their position within the support relationship.

First wave: the road to independence

Campaigns in the late 1970s and 1980s led to calls by disabled people for greater civil rights to live in the community, and led to the now defunct Independent Living Fund, created to allow those with high support needs to pay for their own private care and support. This movement expanded and encompassed local authority social care, where funding could not be made available to disabled people until the passing of the Community Care Direct Payments Act (1996). The act allowed local authorities to make cash payments to disabled people to procure their own PAs. Typically, young, physically impaired, disabled people were at the forefront of the early campaigns and the various policy changes addressed their desire for greater choice and control. The act was further supported by successive governments through the personalisation agenda, which extended independent living to a wider group of service users including people with learning disabilities, mental health users, older people, children and young people and carers.

Initially the practicalities of self-direction were chosen and designed by people living with physical and cognitive disabilities themselves, and were underpinned by an independent living philosophy which places primary importance on the autonomy of disabled people to have overall control over their care and support. This resulted in the development of an approach which saw disabled people as employers of their PAs. This employment relationship was fixed within a legal framework itself underpinned by top-down hierarchies between employer and employee. Many disabled people embraced the idea of being someone's boss and willingly took on responsibility for managing every aspect of their care and support.

Disability literature rarely challenges this top-down relationship between employer and employee. In fact, guidance and support guides published by disabled people and allies (Vasey, 2000; Skills for Care, 2009) perpetuate the idea that disabled people alone are responsible both legally and practically for their PAs.

As a result, increasing numbers of service users oversee their own management, with each service user individually responsible for their own care and support, including the day-to-day supervision of PAs, whom they are both responsible for and in control of. While these shifts have been liberating for many disabled people, the practicalities of these responsibilities are challenging, covering as they do legal, financial, health and safety and logistical management challenges with no professional or infrastructural resources. The next section seeks to explore some of the consequences for service users and the impact for PAs.

Second wave: the reality of independence

While the literature espouses the benefits of increased choice and control (Duffey, 2010), the myriad of official guidance and support documents, policies and procedures pertaining to the oversight and financial monitoring of service user spend (Vasey, 2000; Department of Health, 2011; Skills For Care, 2009) demonstrates the complex processes that individuals are expected to manage. Existing literature focuses on the individual and legal responsibility of the service user, often referred to as the employer, towards their support worker or PA, referred to as the employee. Yet there is little focus on assisting service users to assess the quality of the support in relation to meeting their personal outcomes, and little clarity about the role PAs play in supporting their employers to achieve personal outcomes. An underlying assumption pervades self-direction and personalisation thinking; that service users have complete knowledge of available options and are best placed to deploy rational decision-making in their own best interest, and that providing direction and leadership is an intrinsically desirable state of being. The hierarchical nature of the employer-employee relationship assumes that the direction will come from above; employer to the employee.

From personal experience, employing staff can give satisfaction about being able to actively chose who to employ, but there is no doubt that the potential choices have often been suboptimal and constrained, a factor that the literature often overlooks. The daily reality of managing PAs is isolating, and there is no sidestepping the fact that the employer is legally responsible for their employee. Furthermore, there is an expectation from PAs that their employer alone will instruct them. Managing staff around the clock is a full time job and most days it is a burden. Staff have expectations of you as their employer. This is the price that many disabled people have paid for their independence. In return for being able to get up, go to sleep and bathe when we want and eat what we like, many of us have agreed to take on the responsibility for managing our own affairs as well as taking on the management of PAs.

PAs also report loneliness, isolation and the burden of responsibility of supporting an individual. What if they drop their employer during a transfer out of the bath? What if they tip their employer out of their wheelchair? What if they see their employer doing something risky, is it their place to say something? As it stands, as employees they have little say and are their role is to submit to what is asked of them and not stand in judgement. This means that PAs play no role in providing supervision towards their employer, and the independent living literature is silent on the existence of reciprocity within supervision in the employer-employee relationship.

The literature is also silent on the role social workers have to play in understanding and unpacking whether employers are assessing the quality of support they receive and providing effective and supportive supervision. Reflecting on my personal experience of employing PAs, this conversation has never taken place at reassessments with my social workers. The conversation instead has tended to focus on my personal needs, how those needs are being met and evidence that direct payments are being spent correctly. It is not clear, in any case, that professionals and service users necessarily know or have a common understanding of what good supervision looks like. Furthermore there is no agreed standard for the core skills of PAs, nor is there any clarity about what say personal assistants have about their role and the management they receive. The UK Government, and to a large extent professionals, have delegated these complex issues to service users themselves, usually in the name of service user empowerment.

While social care literature says little about the complexities and burdens of management and supervision, there is evidence in health literature that professionals often delegate responsibility to patients in the form of patient empowerment and involvement (May *et al*, 2009; 2014; May 2005; Kennedy *et al*, 2007). This is often done to alleviate pressures on clinician time, especially where patients have complex long-term health conditions (Gallacher *et al*, 2013). The daily management responsibility is transferred to patients, and research shows that this often results in a treatment burden on patients.

In reality, like all employers and business people, service users procuring and managing their own care are dealing with a large number of issues, including problems with the quality, supply and performance of the workforce, competition, bureaucracy and administrative overload. However, unlike small businesses, a service user cannot risk failure. There are no business support, investment or training schemes for employing staff and all of the legal onus, and therefore risk, lies with the service user.

The questions of how this management can be structured optimally and what good supervision looks like in practice urgently need to be addressed in a sustainable and reciprocal way. A challenge for the independent living philosophy is that, while it seeks to free service users from the oppression of state intervention and professional interference, it simultaneously risks repeating that oppression in the hierarchical relationship it fosters between employers and employees (service users and PAs). If we say we are against being oppressed then how can we participate in management structures which potentially oppress PAs?

In my experience, when the conversation about the training of PAs, pinning down of skills and attributes for being a good PA or for discussing a framework for management and supervision beyond the superficial is discussed, service user groups can feel threatened. Understandably, many service users feel that any attempt to define these skills or develop supervision frameworks pushes PAs into a professional grouping. As such there has been a push back from service user groups because the fear is that the professionalisation of PAs places service users back to being the only non-professionals present, and brings echoes of previous user/professional hierarchies.

In an attempt to alleviate some of these management responsibilities, service user groups have established user-led organisations which provide peer support on management and supervision of personal assistants. These bring people together to share knowledge, experience and expertise on the practical aspects of managing staff and other administrative supports, while alleviating some of the burden involved and arguably have done little to disrupt the hierarchy between employer and employee.

Thus, in practice, the self-directed independence model to some degree perpetuates supervision or 'watching from above' from service users towards their PAs. While sharing experiences with other disabled people is extremely useful, ultimately the individual employer remains responsible for their staff members. The burden of management and supervision continues to rest heavily on the individual's shoulders.

To tackle these issues, six years ago I and a few disabled people wrote a number of accredited training courses for service users opening up the possibility of a market in peer support brokerage services offering management and supervision support to other service users. After critical reflection, this approach is recognised as failing to address structural and conceptual problems, since it repeats cycles of supervisory hierarchy and fails to reverse power differentials. Even when individuals choose to delegate to a support broker, this broker would still be 'watching over' and supervising the PAs, leaving the top down model of supervision merely transferred rather than addressed.

Third wave: beyond independence

Fostering a non-hierarchical supervision approach that addresses the power imbalance between employer and employee demands that we firstly re-conceptualise this relationship and secondly re-conceptualise supervision. This will allow us to consider the skills and capabilities required for the roles. Without addressing these conceptual issues, the burden will always remain with the individual and any attempt to remedy the burden will result in responsibility being transferred and delegated rather than being replaced with more sustainable approaches.

Recent thinking on social work supervision has become more egalitarian (Brookfield 2005; Noble & Irwin 2009), with some move towards a more co-developed relationship, consistent with the influence of feminist theory on social work. Co-developed supervision requires a radical equality between those involved. Miehls (2010) states that this represents a move away from traditional psychoanalytic conceptions of supervision towards supervision that is based on trauma and relational theories. He argues that these more relational theories are underpinned by mutuality, growth and healing which occur within co-created partnerships.

Yet much disability literature and recent social policies, focused on personalisation and self-directed support, continue to perpetuate the hierarchical formulation of service users as managers of PAs, with social workers outside of this supervision relationship (Carr, 2011). Moving beyond this supervisory dyad is important to developing a sustainable and egalitarian approach. Tsui (2005) observed that while the supervisory relationship is often seen as being between supervisor and supervisee, in fact the supervisory relationship goes beyond that and often includes other professionals and agencies. The employer and PA are in fact engaged in a wider supervision dialogue that includes conversations about professionals and agencies even when they are not in the room. Tsui (2005) therefore suggests that the supervision relationship stretches to parties beyond those directly involved and is interconnected and mutually dependent or interdependent.

Since the somewhat loose conceptual underpinnings of supervision have depended on either an institutional view of accountability, in the case of classic supervision, or a moderation view of accountability, in the case of peer or group supervision, the challenge was to explore how mutual accountability could take place between professionals, paraprofessionals, carers and service users.

True mutual accountability requires a radical equality which disrupts all boundaries between practitioner identities and service user identities. Outputs, outcomes, 'professional development' and learning are jointly owned and jointly driven. The concept of individual control, which has dominated the discourse of independent living, dissolves and becomes meaningless. The concept of 'expertise' as locating at an individual level either as 'professional' expertise, or expertise 'by experience', also dissolves as the relational quality of knowledge and therefore growth and success becomes evident. In this approach all goals become interconnected and group-directed. This is entirely distinct from peer group supervision, which, while it has a seemingly flat hierarchy, still focuses on linear professional development and requires independent moderation. The group-directed version could be better described as 'intervision'.

Intervision is by nature disruptive as it challenges roles and identities and requires professionals to reframe their own professional identities and submit to an interdependent group identity. The group's primary objectives may be wildly different to the service objectives and metrics to which the practitioner's employment and training appear to constrain them. Similarly, the service user's self-identity will be radically challenged, when the core objectives they have been told to aim for, namely choice, control and autonomy are revealed to be conceptually flawed and potentially even barriers to interdependence and universal well-being.

Intervision is in many ways underpinned by the relational theories put forward by feminism. It represents a paradigm shift from the individual focused personalisation and self-directed support. Developments in feminist psychology may help us to develop a practical framework for the skills that intervision might include. The relational cultural approach developed by Miller (1968; 1986) is underpinned by a commitment to social justice and human relationships. The approach maintains that human beings are wired to move in the direction of connection and growth-producing relationships, and that individually orientated approaches lead to disconnection, isolation and burden (Eible, 2015). Within the relational cultural approach, relational competence is the goal. Relational competence is demonstrated when there are the following attributes in the relationship:

▶ Movement toward mutuality and empathy.

▶ Openness to influence.

▶ Connection as a priority.

▶ Anticipatory empathy, noticing and caring about our impact on others.

▶ Relational curiosity.

(Jordan *et al*, 2004)

We would suggest that relational competence may provide the anchors needed to develop the competence for intervision, though further research will be required to fully understand how intervision competencies can be supported. In order to move in this direction a group of pioneering disabled people, PAs and social work students, have come together to co-develop intervision in practice in a group called the Interdisciplinary Incubator. This was made possible because this group of people had already made significant strides in pooling their individual siloed budgets together and had included PAs into a co-operative, where they were no longer employed by individuals but by the group working co-operatively with social work students on placements. This new co-operative infrastructure has supported the group to begin to disrupt supervision and co-create intervision.

Conclusion

Intervision represents one of the key drivers to achieving these ends and, we would argue, that it is key to moving from oppressive and burdensome 'personalisation' to an energising 'mutualisation'. This is a journey that many service user groups, personal assistants and professionals have travelled. Our intention in this chapter was to present how we might be able to move beyond the position to which we may have become fixed, to open up a space to disrupt current thinking about how we may become empowered. There are many times more PAs, informal carers and other care paraprofessionals in the UK whose development, involvement and perspective has gone under-researched and under-invested in. We hope that the ideas and innovations presented in this chapter demonstrate the power of bringing about a group-directed support approach to social care. In order to succeed, this approach, which challenges the professional silos which allow power and investment differentials to be permanently perpetuated, requires trialling, peppercorn funding, research testing and some influential proponents.

References

Brookfield S (2005) *The Power of Critical Theory.* Jossey Bass: San Francisco.

Carr S (2011) Enabling risk and ensuring safety: self-directed support and personal budgets. *The Journal of Adult Protection* **13** (3) 122–136.

Department of Health (2011) *A Framework for Supporting Personal Assistants Working in Adult Social Care* [online]. Available at: https://www.gov.uk/government/uploads/system/uploads/attachment_data/file/215508/dh_128734.pdf (accessed November 2015).

Duffy S (2010) The citizenship theory of social justice: exploring the meaning of personalisation for social workers. *Journal of Social Work Practice* **24** (3) 253–267.

Eible L (2015) *Social Work Supervision Through a Relational/Cultural Theoretical Lens* [online]. University of Pennsylvania. Available at: http://repository.upenn.edu/cgi/viewcontent.cgi?article=1062&context=edissertations_sp2 (accessed November 2015).

Evans J (2003) *The Independent Living Movement in the UK.* Available at: http://www.independentliving.org/docs6/evans2003.html (accessed November 2015).

Gallacher K, Morrison D, Jani B, Macdonald S, May CR, Montori VM, Erwin PJ, Batty GD, Eton DT, Langhorne P & Mair FS (2013) Uncovering treatment burden as a key concept for stroke care: a systematic review of qualitative research. *PLOS Medicine* **10** (6) e1001473.

Jordan J, Hartling L & Walker M (2004) *The Complexity of Connection: Writings from the Stone Center's Jean Baker Miller Training Institute.* New York: Guilford.

Kennedy A, Rogers A & Bower P (2007) Support for self-care for patients with chronic disease *BMJ* **335** (7627) 968–970.

May C (2005) Chronic illness and intractability: professional-patient interactions in primary care. *Chronic Illness* **1** (1) 15–20.

May C, Montori VM & Mair FS (2009) We need minimally disruptive medicine. *BMC Health Services Research* **339** (aug11_2) b2803.

May C, Montori VM, Richardson A, Rogers AE & Shippee N (2014) Rethinking the patient: using burden of treatment theory to understand the changing dynamics of illness. *BioMed Central Health Services* **14** (281).

Miehls D (2010) Contemporary trends in supervision theory: a shift from parallel process to relational and trauma theory. *The Clinical Social Work Journal* **38** (4) 370–378.

Miller JB (1968) *Glossary of Relational-cultural Theory Key Terms* [online]. Jean Baker Miller Training Institute website. Available at: http://www.jbmti.org/Our-Work/glossary-relational-cultural-therapy (accessed November 2015).

Miller JB (1986) *Toward a New Psychology of Women* (2nd edition). Boston: Beacon Press.

Miller JB (1988) *Connections, Disconnections and Violations. Work in Progress, No. 33.* Wellesley, MA: Stone Center Working Paper Series.

Noble C & Irwin J (2009) Social work supervision: an exploration of the current challenges in a rapidly changing social, economic and political environment. *Journal of Social Work* **9** (3) 345–358.

Skills For Care (2009) *Exploring Personal Assistants Toolkit* [online]. Available at: http://www.skillsforcare.org.uk/Document-library/Employing-your-own-care-and-support/Employing-personal-assistants-toolkit.pdf (accessed November 2015).

Tsui MS (2005) *Social Work Supervision: Contexts and concepts*. Thousand Oaks, CA: SAGE.

Vasey S (2000) *The Rough Guide to Managing Personal Assistants. National Centre for Independent Living* [online]. Available at: http://www.independentliving.org/docs6/vasey2000.html#1 (accessed November 2015).

Chapter 13

Interprofessional supervision in services to adults: Supervision, outcomes and what next for research and practice

Dr Lisa Bostock

Introduction

This book brings together researchers, practitioners and service users who explore the evidence base for interprofessional supervision and offer new ways of thinking about supervisory approaches that may differ to our own. It challenges us to think about the blurring of boundaries between different professional groups, between professionals and service users, between service users and personal assistants, and what these trends mean for outcomes.

This final chapter reviews some of the key themes, debates and questions discussed during this book. These are situated within the context of a shift toward integrated working, whereby research is encouraged but findings often ignored at the convenience of policy makers and politicians convinced that integration is a 'cure-all'. It explores what supervision means to organisations and their workers, and reminds us that the ultimate purpose of supervision is to improve the lives of people using services. Throughout this chapter, I consider the place of supervision within professional practice before offering some suggestions about where next for research on supervision in adult services.

Integrated working, supervision and the paucity of evidence

In her foreword, Lyn Romeo, the chief social worker for adult social care, acknowledges that supervision has not had enough attention in mainstream social work and social care practice with adults. She describes a sector dominated by the demands of care management, eligibility decisions and process-led approaches to assessment at the expense of person-centered approaches and emphasis on the emotional and social support needs of staff.

It is five years since the then new coalition government introduced the controversial white paper *Equity and Excellence: Liberating the NHS*. This represented one of the biggest shake-ups of the health system since the NHS was established. Integration of health and social care was a central theme. At that time, I was working for the Social Care Institute for Excellence (SCIE) and worked with colleagues to develop a programme of work on integration in services to adults, looking at different aspects of the evidence base for integrated working, including research, practitioner and service user perspectives.

We found the evaluation evidence was less than compelling, largely consisting of poor quality and poorly reported small scale evaluations of local initiatives (Cameron *et al*, 2012). No evaluations that we identified included an analysis of cost effectiveness. When we looked specifically for examples of evaluations of interprofessional supervision, there were too few studies to review. Even when we stepped back and looked more broadly for evidence of effectiveness for supervision in social work and social care, we still concluded that the evidence base was 'surprisingly weak' – most of the studies were correlational and derive from child welfare studies in the US. In other words few addressed supervision in services to adults. No studies attempted to unravel the link between supervision and outcomes for service users and carers (Carpenter *et al*, 2012).

In spite of the shaky evidence base for integrated working, the drive toward integration of health and social care services has gathered pace. In part, this reflects a broad political consensus that care and support should be person-centered, promote independence and be integrated around the needs of the individual. Indeed, both the Health and Social Care Act (2012) and the Care Act (2014) make provision to encourage more integration between services in order to improve quality of care.

In part, it also reflects significant downward pressures on health and social care commissioners to make cost savings, and integration is presumed to be a means to reduce unnecessary duplication across service provision (Chapter 1).

Where integrated working works well, practitioners report positive working relationships, shared learning across disciplines and a more holistic and joined-up service for users (Chapter 10). Where organisational systems and processes militate against integration, multidisciplinary working can prove fractious and difficult to manage, meaning service users might receive contradictory advice about care and support following a joint assessment (Chapter 11). While there is no means of knowing actual numbers of newly integrated or reconfigured services, in practice, from the introduction of integrated health and adult social care teams in Leeds to the Lambeth Living Well Collaborative, which works with people with continuing mental health problems, integrated working requiring interprofessional supervision is an increasingly embedded feature of our care and support landscape.

With colleagues, we have argued that '*the overall aim of professional supervision should be to provide the best possible support to service users in accordance with the organisation's responsibilities and accountable professional standards*' (Carpenter et al, 2012, p.3). This is echoed by Townend (2005) who describes interprofessional supervision as '*Two or more* [practitioners] *meeting from different professional groups to achieve a common goal of protecting the welfare of the client.*' Yet not all supervision takes place between staff employed within health and social care organisations, nor would all service users consider themselves in 'need of protection.' Since the Community Care (Direct Payments) Act (1996), many service users have directly employed personal assistants to support their aspirations of independent living. However, little research has explored this shift of responsibility for procuring and managing support staff from professionals to service users and what this means for supervision across personal and professional boundaries.

This book addresses this gap in our knowledge about supervision across professional boundaries, offering insights and affirmations to practitioners engaged already in this practice with little or no guidance. It is also an opportunity to identify areas for further research, posing questions developed by realist evaluators (Pawson & Tilley 1997); what works for whom in what circumstances, in what respects, and how? Such an approach allows us to move away from binary conditions, whereby interprofessional supervision is 'good' or 'bad', or involvement of service users 'helps' or 'hinders'. It also allows us to explore more systematically the outcomes of different types of supervision in different contexts for different stakeholder groups.

Interprofessional supervision, experiences and outcomes

In our chapter (Chapter 2), Webb, Bostock and Carpenter describe our surprise at identifying such a limited evidence base on the effectiveness of supervision, particularly in relation to services to adults. Of the 50 papers that we identified in our international review of the literature, just 14 focused on adult services. While the majority (10 of 14)

were set in integrated services, only two explore in any detail how supervision operates within a multidisciplinary setting. Davys and Beddoe (Chapter 4) conducted a wider review of the evidence base on interprofessional supervision and included studies focused on the incidence and experience of interprofessional supervision within specific professions. Of the nine studies reviewed, practitioners by and large report satisfaction with this type of supervision, although challenges as well as benefits are explored. While acknowledging the concern that interprofessional supervision can erode professional boundaries, they argue that it also supports professional practice by encouraging '*practitioners to move from their known fields and present their work for reflection and critique to the outside eye*' as a means to increase professional competencies.

In Bogo and Paterson's study (Chapter 3) of interprofessional supervision within addiction and mental health services, practitioners from across professions emphasise the importance of supervision to professional identity and practice, particularly the opportunity to reflect on areas of vulnerability, discuss new as well as existing treatment approaches and access supervisors in crisis situations. With some notable exceptions, what's interesting is that when present, supervision was valued regardless of professional discipline. Indeed, our review showed that satisfaction with supervision is associated with self-reported improved role competence and positive impact on practice.

Yet when reviewing the above chapters, there is a noticeable lack of attention to the social, psychological and emotional functions of supervision, something that was a strong feature in the literature on what makes supervision effective in services to children and families. While elements are discussed, such as the importance of trusting and honest relationships, much is focused on task assistance or improved understanding of different roles and responsibilities. This overlooks the emotionally challenging aspects of the job, whether managing risk and safeguarding people from abuse, supporting people and their families through end of life and bereavement, or working to foster independence and choice within constrained resources. Supervision is an opportunity to explore the impact of emotions on practice and professional judgment, unpacking those that impact negatively and may make staff feel anxious and avoidant. It is also an opportunity to feel supported and looked after, which is essential if staff are to offer a quality service to others. The importance of supervision as a staff support mechanism is a recurring theme of this book.

Delivering compassionate care

As Wallbank discusses in Chapter 7, worker stress, burnout and lack of compassion are frequently associated with the caring professions. High role conflict, what might be called the 'frazzle factor', makes for stressful working environments. Workers experience multiple and competing demands; coping with resource shortfalls, the impact of spending reductions, increased public demand for services and pressure from other agencies. In such conditions, worker capacity to think and show compassion can be compromised. When critical thinking is affected, particularly the ability to revise judgments in the light of new evidence, mistakes are made (Bostock *et al*, 2005) or worse, casual care can become the norm (Francis, 2013).

As a direct response to the fast-paced and emotionally challenging nature of the work, compassion coaching offers the opportunity to be in the moment, *'thereby modeling the kind of quality attention that enables people to thrive – on purpose and without judgment'* (Chapter 8). In this approach, the flow of compassion is emphasised, to oneself, to service user and carers, to colleagues. Listening without judgment is a feature of Schwartz Rounds, which encourage groups of professionals to come together and present their experiences in a safe space, enriching understanding of each others' roles and deepening compassion towards patients and service users, as well as themselves and other professionals. Another approach, restorative supervision, builds the resilience of workers to *'understand their own vulnerability and triggers'* and support them maintain their capacity to think (Chapter 7).

The late Tony Morrison's integrated 4x4x4 model of supervision also stresses the importance of working with emotions by *'valuing intuitive responses and combining these with analytical thinking in order to inform judgments, decisions and plans'*. In Chapter 6 Jane Wonnacott summarises the model that brings together the four main functions, with the four main stakeholders and four main processes of supervision. Where fully implemented, the 4x4x4 model reduces stress and improves worker job satisfaction, retention and effectiveness (Carpenter *et al*, 2012).

Supervision and service user involvement

In Morrison's model, there are only two stakeholders physically present in supervision (the supervisor and supervisee) but it is the job of the supervisor to ensure that other stakeholders, specifically service users, are kept in mind. But what if service users were to be physically present in supervision? What would this mean for the practice of supervision, whether interprofessional or profession specific? What if it is service users doing the supervising, what does this mean for professional boundaries? As Marrable and Lambley note in Chapter 5, the Care Act (2014) sets out service user involvement in decision making as one of the act's key principles, linking it to the personalisation agenda stating:

> '…the importance of the individual participating as fully as possible in decisions about them and being provided with the information and support necessary to enable the individual to participate. Care and support should be personal, and local authorities should not make decisions from which the person is excluded.' (Department of Health, 2014, p4)

Supervision is a primary site of decision making by professionals about risk levels and the care and support needs of individuals, yet service users may not even be aware of its existence, let alone involved to any meaningful degree. Marrable and Lambley conducted two focus groups with service users: the first included 11 people using community mental health services and the other with a group of five adults with learning disability. While small in scale, this study is groundbreaking in terms of asking service users about their knowledge, views and involvement in supervision. They found

that, for the most part, service users had limited knowledge of the supervision process: *'they wanted to know how workers made sure that what service users want, think, and feel is heard within it. They wanted to know how they could be more involved in supervision, as it was concerned with them and their care, but also understood that workers needed to have time with a supervisor to talk about their feelings because "they have to deal with some of our difficult feelings and it can be difficult for them".'*

The suggestion that service users might be more directly involved in supervision may be profoundly uncomfortable for professionals, but potentially beneficial to the development of their practice. Traditional models of professionalism have created too big a gap and power discrepancy between the professional and the person using their service. More equal and complementary ways of working have emerged recently, as Maryam Zonouzi's chapter within this volume illustrates (Chapter 12). She draws on both personal experience as a service user and academic interests to challenge the 'top-down' model of supervision.

Maryam presents an alternative approach to supervision that is group-based and involves professionals, paraprofessionals such as personal assistants, service users and carers coming together to ensure *'all goals become interconnected and group-directed'*. This is not a version of peer supervision whereby professionals come together to offer each other support, rather an attempt to share accountability in a flat hierarchy that transcends boundaries of professional and service user, service user and personal assistant. It radically alters the dynamic of traditional supervision that 'watches over' practice by professionals with service users, or service users with personal assistants and creates a relational approach of 'watching between' service users, personal assistants and professionals.

Concluding thoughts

Changing demography and patterns of illness mean that more of us are living longer with a mixture of multiple and complex needs that Richard Humphries, assistant director at the King's Fund, describes as defying *'organisational boundaries and budgets'* and requiring flexible forms of joint working. At the same time, serial reorganisation means that commissioning responsibilities for different aspects of health and social care are now scattered across 400 separate bodies in the NHS and local government, making the drive toward joined up working more difficult (Humphries, 2015). Such layers of service complexity necessitate skilled supervision often across interprofessional boundaries to ensure that practice remains person-centered and collegiate.

Yet, the international research literature on the effectiveness of supervision is surprisingly limited, particularly in regard to services to adults. While this book addresses the gap in the knowledge base, more evidence is needed to understand whether implementation of different models of supervision does make a difference to outcomes and if so, for whom, in what circumstances and how. This is particularly pertinent in light of both an international shift toward interprofessional supervision, and emerging approaches led by service users. This requires research to identify the structure, frequency and focus of supervision, unpack the impact of professional background, and develop outcome measures defined by service users in conjunction with professionals.

Such research must acknowledge that service user-defined outcomes may differ from policy and practice imperatives. They are a crucial aspect of understanding the effectiveness of services from the perspectives of those who use them, and consequently are important for supervisors to appreciate and for research to investigate. And yet, no study has addressed what service users consider to be the outcomes that matter most from supervision (Carpenter *et al*, 2013). Given the strong commitment in policy, practice and regulation to ensuring effective supervision, research should develop the tools to assess its costs, benefits and cost-effectiveness.

There is much to investigate, from group supervision and 'intervision' to a multitude of cross-disciplinary supervisory relationships in a variety of care and support settings. These include supporting transitions from children's to adult services. It is imperative that we support practitioners and their organisations to make best use of their resources within rapidly changing and confusing systems and constrained resources if we are to provide the best possible support to service users. They, in turn, are now statutorily entitled to be actively involved in decision making, and in some circumstances, are developing their own supervisory approaches which break down barriers between professionals and people using services.

References

Bostock L, Bairstow S, Fish S & Macleod F (2005) *Report 6 Managing Risks and Minimising Mistakes in Services to Children and Families*. Social Care Institute for Excellence (SCIE). London: SCIE.

Carpenter J, Patsios D, Wood M, Platt D, Shardlow S, Scholar H, Haines C, Wong C, Blewett J (2012) *Newly Qualified Social Worker Programme Final Evaluation* (2008 to 2011). Department of Education Research Report DFE-RR229. Available at: http://www.kcl.ac.uk/sspp/policy-institute/scwru/pubs/2012/reports/carpenteretal2012nqswfinal.pdf (accessed November 2015).

Carpenter J, Webb CM, Bostock L & Coomber C (2012) *Research Briefing 43: Effective supervision in social work and social care*. Social Care Institute for Excellence (SCIE). London: SCIE.

Carpenter J, Webb CM & Bostock L (2013) The surprisingly weak evidence base for supervision: Findings from a systematic review of research in child welfare practice (2000-2012). *Children and Youth Services Review* **35** (11) 1843–1853.

Cameron A, Lart R, Bostock L & Coomber C (2012) *Research Briefing 41: Factors that promote and hinder joint working in health and social care*. Social Care Institute for Excellence (SCIE). London: SCIE.

Department of Health (2010) *Equity and Excellence: liberating the NHS*. London: The Stationery Office.

Department of Health (2014) *Care and Support Statutory Guidance Issued under the Care Act 2014* [online]. Available at: https://www.gov.uk/government/publications/care-act-2014-statutory-guidance-for-implementation (accessed November 2015).

Francis R (2015) *Report of the Mid Staffordshire NHS Foundation Trust Public Inquiry: Volumes 1-3*. London: The Stationery Office. Available at: www.midstaffspublicinquiry.com/report (accessed October 2015).

Humphries R (2015) *Putting Social Care in the Vanguard* [online]. ADASS blog post. Available at: http://www.adass.org.uk/putting-social-care-in-the-vanguard/ (accessed November 2015).

Pawson R & Tilley N (1997) *Realist Evaluation*. London: SAGE Publications.

Townend M (2005) Interprofessional supervision from the perspectives of both mental health nurses and other professionals in the field of cognitive behavioural psychotherapy. *Journal of Psychiatric & Mental Health Nursing* **12** (5) 582–588.

Research digest

Research digest

Paul David Spencer Ross

Introduction

The articles contained within this digest cover recently published research studies on interprofessional, social work and clinical supervision, due to a paucity of research in relation to services for adults. Each study listed in this research digest will include a web address to the full research study or abstract including information on how to search for current research on supervision in a variety of settings using a database or search engine. The research abstracts contained within the digest have been arranged into the following four subheadings: research reviews of supervision, studies of interprofessional supervision, peer supervision and profession specific supervision.

Methods

This research digest has been compiled using Social Care Online (SCIE), 'the UK's largest database of information and research on all aspects of social care and social work' and by subject expert recommendations. Additional searches using Google Scholar have been carried out by the author to include clinical settings not indexed in SCIE.

For more information

To find up-to-date research on the subject of interprofessional supervision in adults, visit SCIE using the following keywords 'staff supervision' plus 'adults' in either the basic or advance search.

Research reviews of supervision

Research review of supervision in social work over a forty-year period (1970–2010). This concludes that further research should review the effectiveness of empirically based supervision models and their impact on outcomes for service users.

O'Donoghue K & Tsui M (2015) Social work supervision research (1970–2010): the way we were and the way ahead. *British Journal of Social Work* 45 (2) 616–633. Available at: http://bjsw.oxfordjournals.org/content/45/2/616.abstract (accessed August 2015).

This article is a comprehensive review of the research on the supervision of practicing social workers published in peer-reviewed social work journals over a forty-year period (1970–2010). Eighty-six articles were located and analysed by decade, location, research design, research participants, research focus and findings. Following this analysis, the current state of knowledge is discussed in relation to the foundation it provides for theory and practice in social work supervision. It is recommended that future research efforts should focus on the development of empirically based supervision models, the evaluation of the impact of supervision on client outcomes, as well as comparative cross-national studies on supervision.

Research review of effectiveness of clinical supervision in nursing. The review concludes that there is evidence to suggest that clinical supervision is emotionally supportive, providing stress relief for nurses as well as improving skills and knowledge and promoting professional development.

Brunero S & Stein-Parbury J (2008) The effectiveness of clinical supervision in nursing: an evidenced based literature review. *The Australian Journal of Advanced Nursing* 25 (2) 86-94. Available at: http://search.informit.com.au/documentSummary;dn=253513927962100;res=IELHEA (accessed August 2015)

Objective: Clinical supervision (CS) is attracting attention in the Australian nursing context with efforts underway to embed CS into mental health settings and to extend it to the general nursing population. The purpose of this paper is to review the available evidence regarding the effectiveness of CS in nursing practice in order to inform these efforts.

Method: Relevant literature was located by first accessing research articles in peer-reviewed publications that related to CS and nursing. A total of 32 articles were retrieved. In selecting articles for review, the following criteria were then applied: the article reported an evaluation of the effectiveness of CS; the participants in the study included qualified nurses (not students or generic health care workers); the approach to CS was clearly described; and, the method of data collection and analysis, either quantitative and/or qualitative, was explained in detail.

Results: Of the 32 studies identified in the literature 22 studies met the inclusion criteria. One feature that differentiated the studies was research method, for example, pre-post design; and, articles were initially grouped by method. The reported outcomes of the studies were then categorised according to Proctor's three functions of CS. The results of the studies demonstrated that all three functions, restorative, normative and formative, were evident. The restorative function was noted slightly more frequently than the other two functions. Conclusions: There is research evidence to suggest that CS provides peer support and stress relief for nurses (restorative function) as well a means of promoting professional accountability (normative function) and skill and knowledge development (formative function).

Studies of interprofessional supervision

Empirical study of 243 psychologists and social workers (N = 243) in New Zealand practicing interprofessional supervision. It looks at the rationale for this type of supervision and how it is experienced in practice by supervisors and supervisees alike.

Beddoe L & Howard F (2012) Interprofessional supervision in social work and psychology: mandates and (inter) professional relationships. *The Clinical Supervisor* 31 (2) 178-202. Available at: http://www.tandfonline.com/doi/abs/10.1080 /07325223.2013.730471#.Vdc9mI3bLGI (accessed August 2015).

Supervision of practicing professionals has grown as a major vehicle for the assurance of clinical competence of health and social services professionals in New Zealand with a consequential increase in the demand for competent supervisors. Interprofessional supervision (IPS) has increased as a means of addressing the gap. The literature suggests there is potential for IPS to improve functioning in multidisciplinary teams and enhance clinical work, but it is relatively under-researched. This article reports on a study of psychologists and social workers (N = 243) practicing IPS. The study explored the rationale for seeking IPS and the perceived advantages and limitations for the supervisor and supervisee alike. Professional mandates may limit IPS but its development as a practice suggests that guidance is needed to ensure it meets the aspirations of its practitioners.

Small-scale qualitative study of clinical supervision in three community homes for adults with learning disabilities, using observations and interviews with staff. It explores how clinical supervision was operating, its strengths, its weaknesses and where improvements might be made.

Malin NA (2008) Evaluating clinical supervision in community homes and teams serving adults with learning disabilities. *Journal of Advanced Nursing* 31 (3) 548-557. Available at: http://onlinelibrary.wiley.com/doi/10.1046/j.1365-2648.2000.01309.x/abstract;jsessionid=069C3E590C6B8D856560ED4F6A1236EF.f01t03 (accessed August 2015).

This paper provides a discussion of some of the professional and policy outcomes associated with implementing clinical supervision within a community service for adults with learning disabilities. It is based upon a small qualitative study whose aim was to examine how clinical supervision was operating, its strengths, its weaknesses and where improvements might be made. The study followed the introduction of clinical supervision 9 months earlier for nurses and carers employed in three community homes and one community multiprofessional team. The method consisted of direct observation of individual and group supervision and staff completing critical incident questionnaires, followed by semi-structured, audio-taped interviews with seven registered nurses and four community team members, including a social worker, psychologist and physiotherapist. Outcomes were expressed in two ways: in terms of the benefits of clinical supervision or of its ambivalence. The range of matters brought for discussion, or resolution, in supervision reflected some of the difficulties or dilemmas staff faced working in this area, for example promoting empowerment and assisting clients to make choices, and dealing with clients' challenging and inappropriate behaviours. As for the role of supervisor there was some evidence of nurses expressing apprehension or unpreparedness, also a perceived general concern over the relatively low status of clinical supervision, thought to be due to absence of visible management approval or failure to articulate properly the objective of supervision. A limitation of the study was its small subject sample although considerable data were gathered in each of the units through relatively long-term contact.

Small-scale qualitative study of interprofessional supervision from the perspective of medical and allied heath students on clinical placement. This paper concludes that although participants valued interprofessional supervision, there was agreement that profession-specific supervision was required throughout the placement.

Chipchase L, Allen S, Eley D, McAllister L & Strong J (2012) Interprofessional supervision in an intercultural context: a qualitative study. *Journal of Interprofessional Care* 26 (6) 465-471. Available at: http://informahealthcare.com/doi/abs/10.3109/13561820.2012.718813 (accessed August 2015).

Our understanding of the qualities and value of clinical supervision is based on uniprofessional clinical education models. There is little research regarding the role and qualities needed in the supervisor role for supporting interprofessional placements. This paper reports the views and perceptions of medical and allied heath students and supervisors on the characteristics of clinical supervision in an interprofessional, international context. A qualitative case study was used involving semi-structured interviews of eight health professional students and four clinical supervisors before and after an interprofessional, international clinical placement. Our findings suggest that supervision from educators whose profession differs from that of the students can be a beneficial and rewarding experience leading to the use of alternative learning strategies. Although all participants valued interprofessional supervision, there was agreement that profession-specific supervision was required throughout the placement. Further research is required to understand this view as interprofessional education aims to prepare graduates for collaborative practice where they may work in teams supervised by staff whose profession may differ from their own.

Supervision in a variety of settings

Using a case study approach, this report explores supervision in six social care agencies, including care homes, reablement services and services to adults with disabilities. It identifies 10 learning points including that effective supervision is heavily dependent on the practice context and environment in which it takes place.

Daly E & Muirhead S (2015) Leading change for supervision: messages from practice. Institute for Research and Innovation in Social Services. Available at: http://www.iriss.org.uk/sites/default/files/iriss-supervision-report-100715.pdf (accessed August 2015).

The paper reports on an Institute for Research and Innovation in Social Services (IRISS) projects that explored the topic of supervision with a group of six partners from across the social services sector. The purpose of this report is to share the learning gathered through the project to provide some evidence, inspiration, and pointers for those interested in improving supervision. Key points from the report can be used to prompt reflection and discussion with teams, to review current supervision practice and to help plan improvements.

Each project partner experienced a range of challenges to their plans, however, all were able to make progress, to identify enablers and key learning points. Partner's experiences are explored through five case studies which can be found in section six of the report. The case studies, based on in-depth interviews, provide a snapshot of each partner's context, and detail the challenges and enablers they encountered.

Peer supervision

This paper explores the place of peer supervision, specifically with regard to clinical training and continuing practice development.

Golia GM & McGovern AR (2015) If you save me, i'll save you: the power of peer supervision in clinical training and professional development. *British Journal of Social Work* 45 (2) 634-650. Available at: http://bjsw.oxfordjournals.org/content/45/2/634.abstract?sid=bc36501a-e4f0-4ed1-82db-bb93f33bffc4 (accessed August 2015).

Despite the consensus among practitioners that supervision is a cornerstone of clinical training, comparatively little has been written about the use of peer supervision—particularly in the context of practicum experiences. This article define three kinds of peer supervision: (i) facilitated peer supervision, (ii) planned peer supervision and (iii) ad hoc peer supervision, with an emphasis on the latter. The authors go on to discuss the positive attributes of these practices and their value in the repertoire of clinical training and continuing professional development. In describing how peer supervision can help beginning practitioners, the authors, based on their practicum experiences, provide recommendations on how administrators, directors and supervisors, as well as trainees, can encourage and create opportunities for meaningful peer interaction alongside other, more well-established forms of supervision.

Profession specific supervision

Mixed method study of 636 social workers in Canada, reporting the purpose and duration of supervision, and the training and discipline of supervisors. It identifies some concerns about interprofessional supervision and its impact on professional identity.

Hair H (2013) The purpose and duration of supervision, and the training and discipline of supervisors: what social workers say they need to provide effective services. *British Journal of Social Work.* **43** (8) 1562-1588. Available at: http://bjsw.oxford journals.org/content/43/8/1562 (accessed August 2015).

The intent of this paper is to contribute to an emerging configuration of supervision that has the support of contemporary social workers. A concurrent mixed-model-nested research design was used to discover the post-degree supervision needs of social workers concerning the purpose and duration of supervision, and the training and discipline of supervisors. These four areas of supervision have been investigated and written about repeatedly without resolution. A mixed-methods web survey on supervision was completed by 636 social workers from a broad spectrum of social work practice settings and geographical locations in Ontario, Canada. Quantitative data and written responses from the three open-ended questions are presented as an integrated narrative. The results provide evidence of what social workers say they need as well as their suggestions that could bring ongoing debates closer to resolution. Future research is needed to continue shaping preferred configurations of supervision for effective social work practice.

Longitudinal, mixed methods study of social work supervision practice in the UK. Findings suggest a tapering of supervision for social workers as they become more experienced, but the overall level of supervision appears to be both limited and variable.

Manthrope J, Moriarty J, Hussein S, Stevens M, Sharpe E (2015) Content and purpose of supervision in social work practice in England: Views of newly qualified social workers, managers and directors. *British Journal of Social Work* **45** (1) 52-68. Available at: http://bjsw.oxfordjournals.org/content/45/1/52 (accessed 21 August 2015).

Social work supervision is receiving renewed attention internationally with calls for it to be remodelled and given greater priority, this paper uses data from a longitudinal study in England, which involved: three online surveys of Newly Qualified Social Workers (NQSWs); an online survey of Directors and face-to-face interviews with 23 social work managers which enabled us to investigate the receipt of supervision and its provision. Data on the frequency of supervision were analysed in relation to other job-related factors reported by NQSWs alongside information on NQSWs' views of the content of supervision. Findings suggest a tapering of supervision for social workers as they become more experienced but the overall level of supervision appears to be both limited and variable. NQSWs appreciated supervision from managers, and this affects their engagement with their work. Managers reported pressures of time in providing sufficient supervision. Directors conveyed their perception of the importance of supervision but indicated that there may be blurring of supervision as more structured support for NQSWs becomes part of the requirements for those in their first year in the profession. Greater attention should be given to investigating the effectiveness of supervision and to the support of those managers who are expected to provide it.

Survey of Finnish mental health and psychiatric nurses. Findings demonstrate that efficient clinical supervision is related to lower burnout, and inefficient supervision to increasing job dissatisfaction.

Hyrkäs K (2005) Clinical supervision, burnout and job satisfaction among mental health and psychiatric nurses in Finland. Issues in Mental Health Nursing 26 (5) 531-556. Available at: http://www.tandfonline.com/doi/abs/10.1080/01612840590 931975#.VdM5-43bLGI (accessed August 2015).

This paper presents the findings from a survey of Finnish mental health and psychiatric nurses. The aim of the study was to describe and evaluate the current state of clinical supervision, and ascertain the levels of burnout and job satisfaction experienced by these health care professionals. Clinical supervision was found beneficial for mental health and psychiatric health care professionals in terms of their job satisfaction and levels of stress. The findings seem to demonstrate that efficient clinical supervision is related to lower burnout, and inefficient supervision to increasing job dissatisfaction.

Small-scale study of hospital social work suggesting that supervision is driven by managerial concerns rather than focused on the needs of workers and people using hospital services.

Kadushin G, Berger C, Gilbert C & de St Aubin M (2009) Models and methods in hospital social work supervision. *The Clinical Supervisor* **28** (2) 180-199. Available at: http://www.tandfonline.com/doi/abs/10.1080/07325220903324660#. VdNPJo3bLGI (accessed August 2015).

This is the first qualitative study of the perceptions of hospital-based social work supervisees regarding their hospital supervision. Seventeen social workers were recruited using a national listserv and snowball sampling techniques. According to the perception of the clinical social workers participating in the study, hospital social work supervision is organizationally driven rather than worker-focused. Implications for social work education and research are discussed.

Useful tools and resources

Useful tools and resources

Online tools and resources

Social Care Institute for Excellence (SCIE)

SCIE's guide to effective supervision in a variety of settings is one-stop shop for social care practitioners, presenting key findings, current legislation and examples of what is working well to guide and inform practice.
http://www.scie.org.uk/publications/guides/guide50/

SCIE has also produced a film about how the quality of social work in an integrated mental health setting can be enhanced by complementing line management supervision with clinical and professional supervision.
http://www.scie.org.uk/socialcaretv/video-player.asp?v=supervision03

Care Quality Commission (CQC)

In response to recommendations from the Winterbourne View Serious Case Review, CQC has updated the following supporting information and guidance on what effective clinical supervision should include.
http://www.cqc.org.uk/sites/default/files/documents/20130625_800734_v1_00_supporting_information-effective_clinical_supervision_for_publication.pdf

Local Government Association (LGA)

The LGA has produced the following standards for employers of social workers, including what is expected in terms of supervision.
http://www.local.gov.uk/workforce/-/journal_content/56/10180/3511605/ARTICLE

British Psychology Society (BPS)

The BPS develop resources aimed at psychologists but the principles are relevant to all professionals undertaking supervision. Relevant resources include:

Educational & Child Psychology Vol 32 No 3 September 2015: Supervision
http://shop.bps.org.uk/publications/educational-child-psychology-vol-32-no-3-september-2015-supervision.html

Division Clinical Psychology (DCP) – Policy on Supervision
http://shop.bps.org.uk/dcp-policy-on-supervision.html

Flying start resource for newly qualified staff in Scotland have a learning module on supervision with open access

http://flyingstart.scot.nhs.uk/learning-programmes/safe-practice/clinical-supervision/

Nursing and Midwifery Council (NMC)

The NMC has published the following guides to the supervision of midwives.
http://www.nmc.org.uk/globalassets/sitedocuments/nmc-publications/nmc-standards-for-preparation-of-supervisors-of-midwives.pdf

Royal College of Nursing (RCN)

The following are selected publications on clinical supervision from the RCN and are downloadable from the RCN website.
http://www.rcn.org.uk/development/practice/clinical_governance/staff_focus/rcn_publications#supervision

British Association of Social Workers (BASW)

The following are selected publications on supervision from BASW and downloadable from the BASW website. They include BASW's policy on supervision and a report that looks specifically at supervision of social workers working in multi-disciplinary teams.
https://www.basw.co.uk/theme/?theme=4&category=38

Skills for Care (SfC)

SfC's toolkit to support the assessed and supported year in employment (AYSE) for newly qualified social workers considers the role of reflective supervision and its essential contribution to holistic assessment.
http://www.skillsforcare.org.uk/Social-work/The-assessed-and-supported-year-in-employment-Adults/The-assessor-and-supervisor-toolkit/The-professional-supervisory-relationship.aspx#

SfC have also developed a resource to support people employing personal assistants. This includes a section called 'Managing your personal assistant' which includes material on supervision geared to people using services who are also employers of their own PAs.
http://www.skillsforcare.org.uk/Document-library/Employing-your-own-care-and-support/Toolkit-4.-Managing-(2015).pdf

Research in Practice for Adults (Ripfa)

This resource helps workers identify aspects of good supervision and enables them to develop these aspects in practice.
https://www.ripfa.org.uk/publications-resources/professional-development/93-getting-the-most-out-of-supervision-practice-tool

Books

Wonnacott J (2012) *Mastering Social Work Supervision*. London: Jessica Kingsley Publishing.

Resources from Pavilion

Bradley AD (2014) *The Compassionate Community – a resource for care home managers to place compassion at the heart of caring for residents and their staff teams* (1st edition). Brighton: Pavilion Publishing.
A resource pack for care home managers who are committed to placing compassion at the heart of the care they provide for residents and their staff teams.
Available at: https://www.pavpub.com/the-compassionate-community/

Knapman J & Morrison T (1998) *Making the Most of Supervision in Health and Social Care: A self-development manual for supervisees*.
A support manual for supervisees in health and social care designed to help supervisees understand the process of clinical supervision sessions.
Available at: https://www.pavpub.com/making-the-most-of-supervision-in-health-and-social-care/

Morrison T (2010) *Staff Supervision in Social Care*.
Available at: https://www.pavpub.com/staff-supervision-in-social-care/
In its 3rd edition this best-selling guide brings essential, newly-developed material, while retaining core material covering the fundamentals of good supervision.

Morrison T (2008) *Strength to Strength*.
A training tool for supervisors, trainers and student teachers to prepare supervisees for supervision.
Available at: https://www.pavpub.com/strength-to-strength/

Wonnacott J (2014) *Developing and Supporting Effective Staff Supervision Training Pack*.
A training pack and reader focusing on training supervisors to deliver one-to-one supervision for those working with vulnerable children, adults and their families. Its flexible structure enables trainers to design their own bespoke training programmes.
Available at: https://www.pavpub.com/developing-and-supporting-effective-staff-supervision-training-pack/

Forthcoming

Wallbank S (2016) *The Restorative Resilience Model of Supervision*.
An organisational training manual for building resilience to workplace stress in health and social care professionals.
A training resource based on the sustainable model of professional resilience, to be used in supervision, coaching and supportive sessions across clinical practices.
For more information go to: https://www.pavpub.com/restorative-resilience-model-of-supervision-training-pack/

Wallbank S (2016) *The Restorative Resilience Model of Supervision.*
A reader exploring resilience to workplace stress in health and social care professionals.
This resource allows an organisation to cascade the restorative resilience approach throughout their staff, initially 'training a trainer', who can then pass the knowledge on to any number of supervisors.
For more information go to: https://www.pavpub.com/restorative-resilience-model-of-supervision-reader/

Wonnacott J & Sturt P (2016) *Supervision for Early Years Workers.*
A guide for early years professionals about the requirements of supervision.
This guide provides a framework and support for early years settings and their staff to implement the expectation of the Statutory Framework for the Early Years Foundation Stage, 2014.
For more information go to: https://www.pavpub.com/supervision-for-early-years-workers/